THE WORLD
ACCORDING TO
DICK FRYMIRE, <u>D.B.S.</u>*

Published by   Distributed by
L. H. "Dick" Frymire   LONGSTREET PRESS, INC.
P.O. Box 33   2150 Newmarket Parkway
314 North Chestnut Street   Suite 102
Irvington, Kentucky 40146-0033   Marietta, Georgia 30067

Printed in the United States of America

1st printing, 1989

Library of Congress Catalog Number 88-083930

ISBN 0-929264-19-3

This book was printed by Arcata Graphics Kingsport Press, Kingsport, Tennessee. The text type was set in Century Expanded by Typo-Repro Service, Inc., Atlanta, Georgia. Design by Paulette Lambert. Illustrations by Don Engler. Photos by Marion Hawkins and Ralph Nash.

NOTICE

This publication is not intended in any way to give medical advice of any kind but is written solely to present folklore medical remedies and cures and weather signs only. The author makes no representations of any kind, either expressly or implied, as to the accuracy of the vast majority of the things contained in this volume. Any remedy—from any source—should be employed with caution, common sense and the approval of your physician.

THE WORLD ACCORDING TO DICK FRYMIRE, <u>D.B.S.</u>*

FOLK MEDICINE & COMMON SENSE

Distributed by

LONGSTREET PRESS

HOW I CAME TO FORECAST WEATHER AND DISPENSE FOLK WISDOM

The tree that I use in weather forecasting, a green-leaf variety of the Japanese maple, was set out in 1928. It is thirty feet tall and has a diameter of twenty-eight to thirty inches. Some think it is a Norway maple instead of a Japanese, but it makes little difference because I use all types of trees for forecasting when I travel. The pods (or seedlings) of this particular tree do not fall until the first week of November, two or three months later than normal.

I made my first forecast study in 1966 and have continued since then. The method I use was revealed to me at a baseball convention by an old friend, now deceased. He was the only person with this knowledge and shared it with me confidentially, advising me not to gamble on it and not to divulge any of the information. He also told me that I would have to come up with something to add to this method after thirteen years. To be quite honest, I never thought I would still be at it after thirteen years, but I found it to be a most interesting hobby. I have no idea how long he had been involved in weather forecasting—apparently most of his life.

My friend told me to make a snow forecast by looking at the leaves, pods, bark, limb structure, and tree mold of a specific tree and reading its signs each day in the month of August, omitting August 31.

True to my friend's caution, beginning in the fourteenth year, I added a new "system" to my forecasting. I installed two thermometers—one taking the temperature of the heart of the tree and one taking the outside temperature. In the fifteenth year, I installed another to take the inside temperature and two to take underground readings—one two inches underground and one four inches. I compare all of these temperatures and continue to observe the parts of the tree recommended by my friend. Then, using a formula, I convert these observations into a forecast.

Weather Tree

Visitors are amazed when they see the tree, set out in 1928.

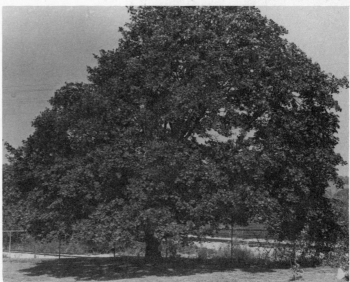

I always preface my forecasts with the warning to "give or take a couple of days" on the dates I give, but I hope eventually to be able to get the forecast to plus or minus twelve hours. To do this will require approximately another ten years of research.

My research was set back as the result of a ransacking of my office on June 29, 1980, when two recorded tapes containing four years of weather data were stolen. A notebook containing my personal coded information on weather data over the past fifteen years was also stolen, in addition to a large United States map and a Kentucky map containing longitude and latitude and elevation identification.

I am the only one in the world with this unique information. I hope one day to pass it on to my son and grandson so that the method will continue to be used.

In addition to the tree formula, I have incorporated other weather forecasting methods, such as:

1) a wind gauge made of a forked stick;

2) a sounding device made of three fifty-five-gallon barrels bolted together; and

3) rain bottles, which are familiar to old-time forecasting enthusiasts.

My studies of weather have enabled me to develop a fishing report that is now carried by several radio stations. The report reveals the best times to fish on any given day. News coverage of my weather forecasting has become nationwide.

Many people have requested information on the rain bottles and weather forecasts. After experimenting with the bottles and a forked stick, I have been successful in predicting short-range forecasts and am happy to pass the information on to you. With the combination of the Mason jar and the Coke bottle (explained below), you will also be able to get good results and maybe avoid a rained-out picnic or two.

To make a homemade barometer, as some people call it, you first have to have a standard quart canning jar, filled with regular tap water to within two inches of the top. Bend two pieces of two-inch-long copper wire and place them over the lip of the canning jar. Then place the Coke bottle (the smaller size) upside down in the jar. After twelve hours the water level should normalize, allowing you to forecast a change in the weather.

The water level inside the Coke bottle is the clue to rain possibilities: the higher the water level, the drier it will be; the lower, the more the chance of rain. Rapid movement inside the Coke bottle indicates severe weather. You should take only about three weeks to get used to reading the "barometer."

To maintain the barometer, you should add water at least once a week. Try not to disturb the water level inside the Coke bottle, or it will take another twelve hours to equalize again. Lift the Coke bottle gently, without taking it out of the water, and pour the new water down the side of the drink bottle. The water should be changed at least once a month.

When the water level indicates approaching rain, then go to the forked stick for further information. The stick I use came from my Japanese maple. It tells me how much rain or snow to expect.

The bottom or base of the stick should be five (5) inches long. The two sides on top should be three (3) inches and six (6) inches. These figures evidently represent the days of the year (365). The ends should be cut off flat.

Use a three-thirty-seconds-inch bit and drill and bore holes as follows:

1) on the three-inch side, drill three holes an equal distance apart, with the first hole directly across from the top of the fork;

2) on the six-inch side, drill six holes, evenly spaced, with the first three-quarters of an inch from the top of the fork;

3) on the five-inch side, drill ten holes evenly spaced, with the first hole being one-half inch from the top of the fork.

Now place the five-inch side into a Coke bottle filled with tap water. (Do not use water that has been run through a water softener.) Never let the bottles stand in sunlight. It will not hurt to disturb the stick.

After the quart jar tells me it is going to rain, I remove the stick from the water. I blow through the holes in the five-inch side to clear them. If they are still stopped up, I count down. Use the following chart to determine the amount of accumulated precipitation:

1) first hole—one-quarter inch;

2) second hole—one-half inch;

3) third hole—one inch;

4) fourth hole—two inches;

5) fifth hole—four inches; and

6) sixth hole—eight inches.

The amount will double as the next hole is stopped up. Once they are stopped up, I use a cotter key to clean them out, and I am ready to start again. This method will take at least six (6) months to catch on to. Replace the stick with a new one every three (3) months.

People from throughout the world have come to see and touch my weather tree. They are generally amazed; some of them try to talk to the tree. It has made Irvington, Kentucky, the Folklore Weather Capital of the World.

On the following pages you will be able to read about folklore weather, but you will also learn much about other kinds of folklore—remedies, cures, signs, sayings—and about old-fashioned common sense. The information included here has been gathered from the wisdom of hundreds of different people who have been kind enough to pass along their knowledge to me. Thousands more have written to confirm that the advice presented here has helped them.

I hope it does the same for you.

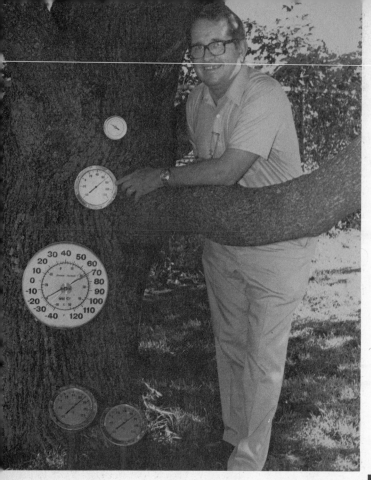

Dick Frymire and His Weather Tree

Note the gauges. The two top ones are taking the temperature of the heart of the tree. The center one is for the outside temperature. The bottom two monitor the soil temperature.

Rain Bottles

The quart jar and the Coke bottle tell when it will rain; the forked stick and the Coke bottle tell how much.

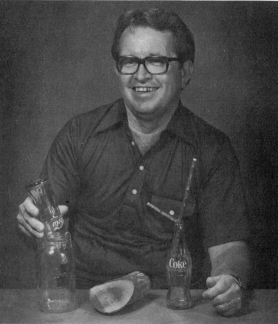

How Ted the Rooster Forecasts

To get Ted to do an economic forecast, the first thing I do is put up an inflation sign with ten grains of corn in front of it. Ted looks at the sign and proceeds to eat the corn. I interpret the number of grains he eats to be the number of percentage points inflation will increase in the next year.

Next I place in front of Ted a tax increase sign with a "yes" and a "no" at its base. Under both the "yes" and "no," I place one grain of corn. The grain Ted eats is his indication about the possibility of a tax increase for the coming year.

I then place a gasoline sign in front of Ted. By this sign, I place two other signs, one with an arrow pointing up and the other with an arrow pointing down. In front of each sign I place one grain of corn. If Ted goes to the arrow pointing down and eats that grain of corn, it means gasoline prices will go down in the coming year. If he goes to the other sign and eats that grain, gasoline prices will go up.

Next I place a stock market sign with two arrows, one pointing up and one down in front of Ted. Again, at the base of each arrow, I place a grain of corn, and Ted predicts the course of the stock market by selecting a grain to eat. If he eats first one grain and then the other, I take that

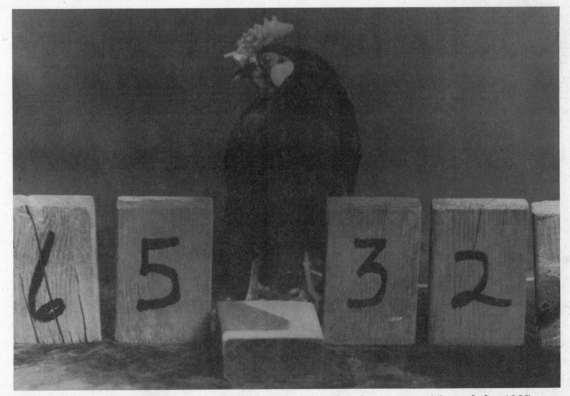

Ted the Rooster, better known as "Derby Ted," picks the post position of the 1985 Kentucky Derby winner.

to mean that the market will go in one direction first, then reverse to the other.

Ted also predicts the unemployment rate. If he eats nine grains of corn, for instance, from under an unemployment sign, this means that the rate for the coming year will be 9 percent.

Finally, I place an old political campaign poster used in the last election in front of Ted. If Ted looks the sign over and begins to crow and flap his wings, I take this to mean that our good brothers and sisters in Washington will again put on a good show for us.

Ted can also predict the outcome of sporting events. For instance, he picked the winner of the December, 1985, University of Kentucky-University of Louisville basketball game. I set up two signs, one with UK Wildcats on it and the other with UL Cardinals. These were placed in Ted's pen. At the base of the signs, I placed twenty grains of corn.

At this point, Ted went straight for the UK sign and nodded his head up and down. He then ate five grains of corn. I took this to mean that UK would win by five, and that's exactly how it turned out.

The UK versus UL game in 1984 was forecast in the same way. Ted picked UL by seven, and that was the margin of their victory.

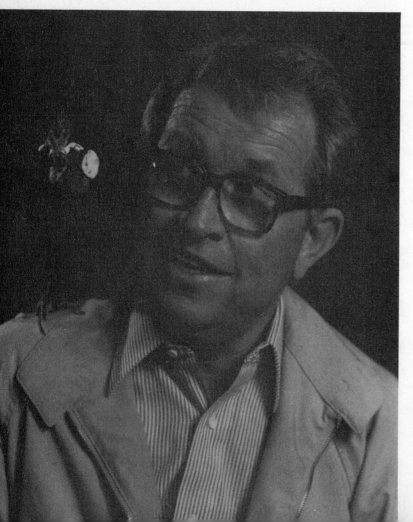

Ted and Dick confer
on Super Bowl results.

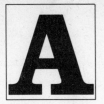

ACNE — If you are bothered with acne, lay off the sweets, soft drinks, cigarettes, and drugs, even prescription drugs. Eat plenty of fresh fruits and vegetables, eggs, and lean meats (especially liver). These foods contain not only vitamin A, but also vitamins B, C, and E. It is also very important to get plenty of sun on your skin.

Rub the affected area with a camphor stick.

Eat three almonds (the sweet variety) daily.

Eat a high-fiber diet.

Eat plenty of alkaline-reacting foods, such as green vegetables and vegetable juices, citrus fruits and their juices, fish, fowl, lamb, whole-wheat bread and whole-grain cereals, and milk. Avoid pork, red meat, fried or greasy foods, chocolate, starchy sweets, white bread, and white potatoes.

Drink one-quarter cup of fresh potato juice twice daily.

Mix one-quarter cup of sugar with one quart of water. Next, lather hands with a mild soap. Dip a part of each hand in the sweet water. Massage the face with this mixture of mild soap and sugar water.

Some people like to lather both hands with soap and then sprinkle on some sugar. Rub the hands till sugar is dissolved and then massage the face. Rinse with lukewarm water and pat dry. Do this twice daily for two weeks. It should start to work by then. Then apply once daily.

Peel an orange and rub the inside of the peel where the acne is. Leave on for thirty minutes. Wash off with a very mild soap. Rinse and pat dry. Do this twice daily.

Try taking fifty milligrams of zinc a day.

Acidophilus also seems helpful in clearing up acne.

One yeast tablet after every meal should clear up your acne.

Rub vitamin-E oil over the affected area. Then apply egg white. Rinse off with clear water. This should do wonders for your face.

Steam your face five minutes over hot water. Then apply a mixture of equal parts fresh heavy cream and fresh cod liver oil. Leave on for a few minutes and then gently wash it off.

ACNE (SCARS) — To help remove, combine one teaspoon of honey with one teaspoon of powdered nutmeg and apply to the scarred area. After the mixture has been on for thirty minutes, wash off with cool water. Do this three times a week.

A

AGE (GUESS) — You can guess anyone's age provided he tells you how much change he has in his pocket. Give him a pencil and paper and ask him to: 1) write down his age; 2) multiply it by two; 3) add five; 4) multiply it by fifty; 5) subtract 365 from the number so obtained. Now ask him for the number as well as the amount of change he has in his pocket less than a dollar. To the number he tells you, add 115 plus the amount of change. Now, if he hasn't made mistakes in arithmetic, the first two digits of the number will be his age and the last two digits will be the amount of change in his pocket.

AGE (SPOTS) — Eat foods high in zinc, such as liver, oysters, red meat, and shellfish. Check with your doctor about zinc supplements.

ALCOHOL (BREATH) — Chew parsley or a piece of orange peel.

ALCOHOL (CLEANER) — Soaps and cleaners are useless on sticky plastic-coated shelves. Wipe the racks with a cloth dipped in rubbing alcohol.

ALCOHOLISM — Try doing without sugar. Your diet should be almost 100 percent protein.

Eat a high-fiber diet.

Eat raw vegetables, such as celery, lettuce, tomatoes, and carrots, as well as cooked vegetables.

Eat fish, fowl, and lamb. Avoid beef.

Go to the ocean or beach and have someone cover you with sand up to your neck. Place a shade over your head. Stay covered for two hours daily.

ALE (RHUBARB) — Combine six cups of rhubarb and one-half cup of sugar. Heat until the sugar is dissolved. Cool and add one-third cup of orange juice, four tablespoons of lemon juice, and four cups of ginger ale. Serve with ice.

ALFALFA — Alfalfa seeds are easy to sprout, and they are very high in protein. They also contain phosphorus, iron, potassium, and vitamins A, E, K, B_8, D, and U. They are also rich in calcium.

ALLERGIES — There are some who believe that many hard-to-explain symptoms can be traced to allergies. Most of the chronic people that doctors can't find anything wrong with have allergy problems, especially with food, and doctors don't recognize it.

To treat allergies, fill a quart jar half full with white raisins. Next, add one pint of gin. Shake two or three times daily for three days. Take the following dosage daily: one teaspoon first thing in the morning on an empty stomach.

What in the world do raisins soaked in gin have to do with allergies and rheumatism? Raisins are covered with mold. When atmospheric conditions change before a rain, molds proliferate, aggravating many types of allergies and related aches and pains.

If you take a teaspoon of these raisins every morning, it's like an oral dose of molds that neutralize — or hyposensitize — the molds in your body. It has nothing to do with the raisins, except the mold on them. Nothing to do with the gin, really. It's what's in it. Caution: Don't try this if you are on any medications.

Do not use anything aluminum to cook with. Use cast-iron skillets.

Many migraine headaches seem to be triggered by allergies.

If you suffer from allergies, do not drink alcohol. Alcohol can speed up an allergic reaction.

Grow as much of your own food as possible or buy from local growers who do not use as many insecticides and chemicals.

Avoid using plastic containers for food storage; always try to use glass containers.

If you are allergic to nylon hose, wash your hose thoroughly. Soak them in a strong vinegar solution for four hours. Drip dry, then wash.

To reduce allergies in children born to parents with allergies, the mother should avoid all foods to which she is allergic during the last three months of pregnancy, and she should breast-feed for the first year, avoiding all foods to which she is allergic.

Solid foods should be introduced to children on a rotation plan to make reactions more visible and identifiable.

ALOE — The juice of a cut leaf soothes insect bites and minor burns. Aloe juice is also good for baldness, wrinkles, and poison ivy rash. Rub on infected area.

ALUMINUM FOIL — This makes very good mulching material and can be used for insect control.

ANEMIA — Try the ginseng tea remedy.

Eat a high-fiber diet.

Eat fresh vegetables, liver, seafood, and whole grain bread.

Drink citrus juices and milk.

Avoid white bread, fried foods, and carbonated drinks.

Massage the spine area with olive oil or peanut oil.

Drink eight ounces of pure grape juice with no sugar or preservatives every day.

Eat two or three dried apricots after breakfast and after supper.

Eat a lot of raw spinach.

ANGINA PECTORIS — Raising the head of your bed ten inches can relieve the heart of some of the strain of circulation. Cold can worsen angina attacks, so dress warmly and in layers in cold weather. Protect your head especially, since most body heat escapes from it. Avoid going out in cold weather and avoid strenuous activity in the cold.

ANIMAL REMEDIES — Cod liver oil may help lameness in horses.

Give brewer's yeast to your horses two or three times a week to keep them free of flies.

If your parakeet is looking droopy, try giving him some sunflower seeds and some liquid vitamin C in his water.

ANTS — Do ants invade your kitchen? If so, attach flypaper—sticky side out—along the bottom of the cabinets (or around table legs) to form an impenetrable barrier. These social little insects will soon realize they are not wanted.

Spray with vinegar to get rid of ants.

Put red pepper in the places ants frequent most.

A small bag of sulphur kept in a drawer or cupboard will drive ants away.

Red ants may be banished from the pantry by strewing the shelves with a small quantity of cloves. The cloves should be renewed occasionally; after a time they lose their strength and decay.

Scrub shelves or drawers with a strong carbonic soap.

Saucers of olive-tar set where ants are will drive them away.

Rub shelves with gum camphor. Two applications one week apart will be sufficient.

Track the ants to see where they are getting in and squeeze the juice of one lemon into the holes and/or crack. Then slice up the lemon and put the peeling all around the entrance.

To get rid of red ants, use sprigs of wintergreen or ground ivy. Use wormwood to get rid of black ants.

Pour household ammonia down the center of an ant hill. You could also make a circle around the hill and fill it with ammonia. Use plenty, about one and one-half cups.

The most effective nontoxic control is boiling water. It works best on cool, sunny days, when ants gather near the tops of mounds. For the best results, open the mound with a shovel and wait until the ants swarm out before pouring on at least a gallon of hot water. A second dousing may be needed.

Wipe or spray with full-strength vinegar on any surface that can't be harmed by the acidic liquid.

Place cinnamon sticks around the outside and inside of your house.

Sprinkle ground cinnamon in cracks around and in your house.

Dust ground black or cayenne pepper where ants travel.

Place cucumber peelings where ants travel. Replace with fresh peelings as the original peels dry up.

Mix one-quarter cup of sugar and one-half cup of sorghum molasses with one package of dry yeast. Place this mixture in small lids and place the lids where ants have been spotted.

Dust powdered cleanser where ants travel.

For those outdoor ants, try this: pour a cup or two of grits near the anthill.

If there are two anthills, dig a shovelful of ants from each one and exchange them by placing the ants from one anthill in the other.

APPENDICITIS – To help prevent appendicitis, start now with a high-fiber diet. Mix one tablespoon of wheat bran with juice and take the mixture twice daily. As time goes on, increase the amount of bran until you are regulated. In some cases you will need to decrease the amount of bran. You will be able to tell.

For appendicitis in the mild to acute stages, you will need to be on a light diet until the discomfort subsides. Eat grapes and drink grape juice; also drink other fruit and vegetable juices. Avoid fried foods and pork.

Apply castor oil packs, without heat, and leave on for five hours.

Apply Epsom salt and grape poultices without heat. The grape poultices should be made by crushing Concord grapes and placing them at least a half-inch in thickness between pieces of cloth. The poultices should be left on for two hours a day, with one change of the poultice during that time.

Use grain alcohol to massage the spine if you have a temperature.

APPLES – For that extra something in your apple pie, sprinkle the sliced apples with a few drops of lemon juice. Do this, and that first apple won't be brown and soft by the time you peel the fifth one.

Place peeled apples in a basin of cold, slightly salted water until you are ready to use or serve them.

A few apples in the potato bin are supposed to keep the potatoes from sprouting.

ARTERIES (HARDENING) – Eat some raw potatoes three times a day.

Drink one cup of warm apple cider thirty minutes before bedtime.

Eat a high-fiber diet.

Massage with olive oil.

Try the Fry-Hut Relaxer (see page 149).

Mix one teaspoon of apple-cider vinegar with eight ounces of water. Take three times daily.

ARTHRITIS — Keep away from things that oversupply your system with salt — limes and the like. Eat foods that carry iron, iodine, and phosphorus to the system.

One meal each day eat citrus fruits, figs, prunes, and berries. Do not eat apples or bananas.

One meal should consist of nuts and the oil of nuts.

One meal should be of well-balanced leafy vegetables. At this meal, eat turnips, eggplant, green vegetables — lettuce, celery, spinach, mustard greens, etc. (no cabbage). The meats should be wild game, fowl, fish, oysters, or other seafoods.

Take three drops of Atomidine in water morning and night. Each day increase the amount one drop until at least ten drops are being taken twice a day; stop for five days, then begin the cycle again.

After forty-five days start taking Epsom-salt baths once a week. Add three to ten pounds of the salt to sufficient water to cover the body up to the neck in the bathtub. The water should be as hot as the body can stand. As it cools, add more hot water. Soak for at least thirty minutes.

After the bath, your body should be rinsed off in plain water, then rubbed dry; next massage thoroughly over the entire body a solution with equal parts of olive oil, tincture of myrrh, and Russian white oil. Heat the olive oil first, then add an equal amount of tincture of myrrh while the olive oil is hot. While the mixture is cooling, stir in an equal amount of the Russian white oil. None of these can be of a paraffin base. They must have been purified. Massage in thoroughly, then rub off with alcohol. Now rest. Use this treatment for four weeks.

Take one-half teaspoon of olive oil three times a day for ten days. Stop for ten days, then repeat.

Massage the bottoms of the feet, under the knees and the spine, and below the kidneys during the menstrual period with the following: five ounces of denatured alcohol to which you have added one ounce of oil of cedar, one ounce of witch hazel, one-half ounce of oil of sassafras, and one ounce of Russian white oil.

Take Epsom-salt baths once a month for three months, then once every ten days. While in such a bath, massage the bottoms of your feet, knees, and muscles both above and below the knees.

Once a week apply Epsom-salt hot packs to the knees. Follow this with a massage using olive oil or peanut oil. Then take four drops of wheat oil three times a week. Follow this with proper diet and rest.

Eat raw carrots, celery, and lettuce. This combination should be mixed and eaten as the greater portion of one meal each day.

Eat cooked cereals, not dried cereals.

Drink grapefruit juice.

Eat fish, fowl, or lamb at least once a week.

Drink red wine as a stimulant.

Soak coarse brown paper in apple-cider vinegar and wrap around the affected joint or joints. Keep this on for at least thirty minutes, three times a day, for ten days. Coarse brown paper from grocery sacks will work fine.

Mix one tablespoon of vinegar and one tablespoon of honey with eight ounces of water and drink with each meal. If you can't take the honey, take the vinegar.

Rub sore joints with castor oil before putting on hot compresses.

Drink tea made from either the seeds or leaves of alfalfa.

Soak a cloth in a mixture of two teaspoons of garlic powder and two cups of vinegar. Apply to the affected joint twice a day for ten days, then once a day thereafter. Each treatment should last at least twenty minutes.

Lay off sweets, colas, and cigarettes.

Eat one-quarter cup of dried raisins once a day.

Eat five almonds each day.

Drink milk or eat yogurt each day.

Eat greens at least twice a week.

Apply moist heat.

Eat a high-fiber diet.

Observe good posture rules.

Drink eight glasses of water a day.

Avoid emotional upsets, tensions, and shocks.

Eat onions.

Season your food with garlic.

You need a balanced mixture of rest and exercise. This may vary, depending on how severely the disease is attacking. There will be more resting and less exercising during an acute stage and vice-versa during improved stages.

Do not get overweight.

Beware of quacks or any advertised "cure" for arthritis—these will waste your money for sure. See a good medical doctor who specializes in the treatment of arthritis. A good understanding between doctor and patient is very important.

Don't rush. Take your time.

Drink a glass of string-bean juice daily.

Mix and shake well the following: one pint of crude oil, one-half pint of turpentine, one-half pint of strong vinegar. Rub this mixture on morning and evening.

Soak in a solution of *yerba la vibora* (turpentine weed).

Mix one part pokeroot tea with eight parts 100 proof whiskey. Take one teaspoon every four hours.

Eat ten cherries and drink a glass of cherry juice daily.

Take two teaspoons of apple-cider vinegar in a glass of water each morning to help battle arthritis pain, high blood pressure, and sleeplessness.

Using one tablespoon of soybean lecithin (granules), one tablespoon of debittered yeast, one tablespoon of raw wheat germ, and one tablespoon of bone meal as your basic proportions, mix up a large batch and store in a dark place. Each morning mix two tablespoons of this mixture with one tablespoon of dark brown or raw sugar and one tablespoon of safflower or soybean oil in a bowl. Dissolve this mixture in milk. You can add plain yogurt to improve consistency. Mix with cold cereal or oatmeal, porridge, or any hot cereal. Raisins and fruit can also be added. If you are a bacon-and-eggs person, mix with homemade tomato juice, leaving out the sugar, and spice the mixture with black pepper or Worcestershire sauce, as the bone meal gives it an unpleasant taste. Drink before eating breakfast.

Try calcium or bone meal tablets.

Some recommend taking calcium and vitamin D combined.

Take six alfalfa tablets a day.

One person claims that by drinking one quart of orange juice a day, her arthritis was cured.

Make a tea out of the blossoms, stems, and leaves of alfalfa plants. They will need to be dried before you make the tea.

Cut a fresh clove of garlic and rub it on the painful area.

Make a poultice of three tablespoons of horseradish and one-half cup of boiled milk and apply to the painful area.

To get rid of the twinges that sometimes accompany arthritis, add to your bathwater the petals of three or four roses that are about to wither.

Steep one cup of parsley in a quart of boiling water for fifteen minutes. Strain and refrigerate. Drink one-half cup before breakfast, one-half cup before dinner, and one-half cup when the pain is severe.

Dice two cups of unpeeled potatoes. Boil them in five cups of water in a non-aluminum pan until only half the water is left. Bathe painful parts of the body with this water while it is still hot, but not scalding.

Heat coarse salt in a skillet and make a poultice out of it. Apply to the painful area.

Take two small capsules of cod-liver oil each morning.

ARTICHOKE (JERUSALEM) — This American variety of the sunflower is a small tuberous vegetable that looks like fresh ginger, crunches like a carrot, tastes sweet and nutty, and has fewer calories than a potato. These have been used as an alternative to insulin.

ASPARAGUS — Wilted asparagus will come to life if the stems sit for a while in cold water.

ASTHMA — Get some ginseng leaves; dry and powder them. Put the powder in a pan, place a hot coal on top of it, then inhale the smoke.

Cheddar cheese might help. One of its ingredients — tyramine — apparently helps to open up the breathing passages.

Drink willow-bark tea.

A child with asthma who wheezes at bedtime will stop and get a good night's sleep if he or she gets a tablespoon of corn oil. In adults, the mixture will decrease the wheezing by 50 percent when it is taken at bedtime. Corn oil, furthermore, if applied to the eyelids at bedtime as one applies an ointment, will favorably influence granulation.

Try not using fabric softener in your washer.

Line-dry all clothes.

Eat five apricots a day.

Inhale the steam from boiling potatoes.

Cut out the salt in your diet.

Eat a piece of raw potato five times daily.

Eat some raw cucumber each day.

Chew on some honeycomb each day.

Drink some buttermilk each day.

Put four cups of sunflower seeds in two quarts of water and boil until only half of the water remains. Strain. Add one pint of honey and boil to a syrupy consistency. Take one teaspoon one-half hour after each meal.

Take one teaspoon of grated horseradish mixed with one teaspoon of honey every night before bed.

Slice up two large onions and place them in a jar. Add two cups of honey, close the jar, and let stand overnight. Take one teaspoon of the "honion" syrup one-half hour after each meal and before bed.

Simmer three peeled garlic bulbs in two cups of water in a non-aluminum pan. When the garlic becomes soft, remove it and put it in a jar. Then add one cup of cider vinegar and one-quarter cup of honey to the water in the pan. Boil until syrupy. Pour over the garlic and let stand overnight. Take one or two cloves of garlic with a spoonful of syrup every morning on an empty stomach.

Drink cranberry juice. Drink two tablespoons one-half hour before each meal and at the onset of an asthma attack.

Some asthmatics have claimed that coffee provides relief from an asthma attack: two cups of coffee may provide relief for a person weighing one hundred to 125 pounds.

I have come to the conclusion that asthmatic attacks could be brought on by spinal problems, diet, and stress. Any one of the three would be enough to do you in. What can be done? Try the following:

Make sure that there is nothing wrong with your back.

Avoid sweets or foods containing sugar.

Avoid beef, fried foods, and large amounts of starches.

Eat mainly vegetables, fruits, and seafood.

Avoid constipation and any blockage of the kidneys.

Drink plenty of water.

Include raw vegetables in at least one meal each day.

Try to relax and forget your troubles.

Mix one tablespoon of wheat bran with one cup of juice and take twice daily. This should get you regulated.

Remember this: keeping your internal pipes in good working order is very important. You are in big trouble if you don't do this.

ATHLETE'S FOOT — Small cotton balls soaked in raw honey and placed between infected toes seems to help. Dab with vinegar morning and night. Dab with vitamin E twice a day.

Wash feet twice a day with soap and water and change socks. Always change your socks once daily or, even better, twice. Use lightweight cotton socks.

Walk barefoot or wear open sandals as much as possible.

Apply talcum powder, baking soda, or lamb's wool between the toes after drying them.

Never wear the same pair of shoes two days in a row and wear leather shoes, which allow the feet to breathe.

Have your butcher trim the fat from around the kidney of a lamb. Remove all the skin and any blood vessels. Cook the fat over a slow fire. Strain the liquid and apply to the feet sparingly after washing.

Soak the feet in a solution of warm salt water and Absorbine, Jr.

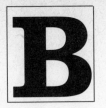

BABY (BABY FOOD THAT CAN BE DIGESTED WHEN ALL ELSE FAILS) — Put one teacup of oatmeal in two quarts of slightly salted boiling water. Let it cook two and one-half hours. Strain. When the mixture is cool, mix one-quarter pint of it, one-quarter pint of thin cream, and one teaspoon of sugar. To this mixture, add one pint of boiling water. The food is now ready to be served to the baby.

BABY (POTION TO AID IN RESTING) — Give the restless baby one-half teaspoon of catnip tea.

BACK PROBLEMS — Moist heat is the best treatment for back pain. Soak a towel in hot water, wring it out, and place it on your back, being careful that it is not too hot.

Twenty-minute baths in warm water, not extremely hot, are helpful.

An ice pack is good for muscle spasms.

Exercise to strengthen the back and abdominal muscles will help prevent future back problems. Brisk walking for about two miles and swimming are two good ways to strengthen back muscles.

Be sure to sit in a firm, comfortable chair and sit back. Keep your knees bent and never cross your legs. Change positions and move around at least once an hour.

If you stand for long periods of time, alternate your weight from foot to foot or elevate one foot.

Sleep on a firm mattress on your side with your knees bent when possible. Never sleep on your stomach.

When you lift, bend from the knees, not the waist. Improper lifting causes most back injuries.

Buy shoes that support your back properly with heels one-half inch or lower.

Wear loose, comfortable clothing, and if you are overweight, you need to reduce.

Soak a cloth in warm apple-cider vinegar and apply the cloth to the sore spot. Place a warm towel over this cloth. Leave on for thirty minutes. Do this three times a day for ten days, then once a day thereafter. After thirty days, you need to apply warm castor-oil packs in the same way.

Try this exercise: Stand up, bend over slightly, relax your arms and hands. Slowly swing your arms crosswise in front of you. Now start bending your back more and at the same time keep swinging your arms. Relax and do this for two minutes.

Apply Epsom-salt packs to relieve back pain.

BAKING (HINTS) — When you are baking a cake, grease the pan and coat it with sugar instead of flour. Your cake will not be burned or scorched.

Use old metal ice-cube trays in baking. They are an excellent size and shape for long, layered loaf cakes.

Use vinegar in the dough for a pie crust instead of water to ensure an always flaky crust.

Do you know how much batter to use in an odd-sized cake pan? Fill the pan with water. You'll need half that amount of batter.

Good flour, when squeezed in your hand, will retain the shape given by the pressure.

BALDNESS — Make a paste by mixing one teaspoon of rubbing alcohol with one teaspoon of Vaseline. Apply this paste to the scalp twice a week for five weeks. Put on at bedtime and leave on overnight. In about three months, the hair will come in thicker.

Take one drop of Atomidine each morning for five days. Leave off for five days and repeat.

Mix one jigger of vodka with one-half teaspoon of cayenne pepper and rub the mixture on the scalp.

Make a tea with peach-tree leaves and rub on the scalp.

Massage the scalp with a mild solution of ammonia once a day, three minutes each time for thirty days. Some have claimed that this made their hair grow. If it is going to work, it will start during the first thirty days.

Dampen the scalp with a mild solution of sulphur water four times a week.

Eat onions.

Eat almonds.

Break a section of grapevine. Set it in a bottle and let the juice drain. Rub the juice on the scalp. Massage the scalp for at least three minutes once a day for twenty days. This treatment should start to work within twenty days.

After drying them, cut twenty to twenty-five dandelion roots into one-quarter-inch pieces. Place these in a pan with one pint of water and let the mixture simmer over a hot fire for fifteen minutes. Do not boil. Drain off the dandelion tea. Massage the scalp with this tea twice a day for ten days. Be sure to massage for three to five minutes each treatment.

Slice one or more medium onions into one-half-inch pieces. Soak these onions in apple-cider vinegar for three days. You are now ready for treatments. Rub these onion slices on the entire bald head for two minutes, three times a day, for ten days. Then once a day for the next twenty days, then once every ten days. Let the mixture dry on the head for at least ten minutes. Wash your head after each treatment with a very mild soap. Pat dry. Be sure you rub or massage your scalp with the onion slices at least two minutes each treatment. This remedy seems to work best of all the folklore treatments.

Promote the growth of hair by applying the following mixture twice a day. Take four ounces of wild indigo, and steep it for about ten days in a pint of alcohol and a pint of hot water. The head must be thoroughly washed with the liquid, morning and evening. Apply with a sponge or a soft cloth.

Mix three ounces of castor oil with just enough alcohol to cut the oil. Then add twenty drops of tincture of cantharides and two drops of perfume. This will soften, invigorate, and strengthen the roots of the hair.

Mix one pint warm water with two tablespoons of soda and five drops of iodine. Apply to the scalp and massage for three minutes, three times a day for ten days, then once a day for ten days. After each treatment, leave the mixture on for fifteen minutes. Wash with a very mild soap. Pat dry. If this treatment is going to work, it will do so within twenty days.

Mix one pint of warm apple-cider vinegar with one teaspoon of honey and five drops of iodine. Massage the scalp with this mixture for three minutes, twice a day for ten days, then once a day for five days. Leave the mixture on the scalp for fifteen minutes. Then wash the head with a very mild soap. Pat dry. This mixture will work within fifteen days if it is going to be successful.

Eat a high-fiber diet.

Always use a very mild soap to wash the scalp.

Drink apple cider at least once a day.

Cut down on your smoking.

Massage the gel of an aloe plant on your head twice a day for eighty days, then once a week.

Massage the scalp with pure crude oil (just as it comes from the ground) for twenty minutes. Rinse out using a 20-percent pure grain (not rubbing) alcohol solution. Wash the scalp using equal parts of olive oil and pure Castile shampoo. There are some who use Vaseline instead of crude oil.

Massage the scalp with hog lard.

Eat cooked peelings from Irish potatoes or drink the water in which peelings have been cooked.

Eat seafood.

Eat raw vegetables and citrus fruits.

Eat plums and figs.

With a mild shampoo, apply quinine, then wash your head.

BANANA BREAD — Did you realize that when you make banana bread, the riper the bananas, the stronger the bread's flavor?

B

BARLEY — Drink barley water every day. It's rich in iron and vitamin B, and it will help prevent hair loss and tooth decay, improve fingernails and toenails, and help heal ulcers, diarrhea, and bronchial spasms. Barley water is also good for chapped skin and sunburn.

To make barley water, boil two ounces of barley in six cups of water until only half of the water remains. Strain. Add honey and lemon to make it more pleasing to the taste.

BASEMENT DAMPNESS — Keep a fan running in the basement to prevent dampness. The fan must be turned toward a window, which must be left partially open.

To test for basement dampness, attach a small mirror to one of the basement walls. Leave it there for eight hours, and if condensation is causing the problem, tiny drops of water will form on the mirror. You can also lay a rubber mat on the bare concrete floor. Leave it for twenty-four hours. If the floor is damp when the mat is removed, that indicates that moisture has penetrated the concrete from below.

BASIL — The strong scent of basil is an aid to meditation and repels insects. Basil tea may relieve certain types of headaches.

BATHING (RULES) — Don't bathe within two hours after a meal.

Avoid bathing when tired.

Don't bathe when the body is cooling after perspiring.

Avoid bathing in the open air if, after having been in the water for a short time, your hands and feet feel chilled and numb.

Bathe when the body is warm. Waste no time getting into the water.

Avoid chilling the body by sitting or standing undressed on the banks or in boats after being in water.

Don't stay in water too long; get out when there is the slightest feeling of chill.

The strong may bathe early in the morning on an empty stomach. The young and weak had better bathe two or three hours after a meal; the best time is two to three hours after breakfast.

Those who become giddy or faint or suffer from palpitation or other heart discomforts should not bathe without first consulting their medical advisor.

BEADS — Don't risk losing your beads because the string breaks. Restring beads on dental floss. The beads will be safe and will hang gracefully.

BEANS (BAKING) — Soak beans overnight and boil as usual. Put the beans, salt, and a tablespoon of molasses in a quart pot. Cover with milk (be sure to use a quart pot, as the milk boils over easily) and refill as the milk cooks away. Bake slowly for nine to ten hours. People with weak digestive systems can eat these beans without harm.

B

BEAUTY TREATMENTS — Wash and massage with buttermilk.

If you are bothered with clogged pores, wash with stone-ground cornmeal twice a day. Apply pure raw liquid honey to your face and neck. Leave the mixture on for twenty minutes, then wipe off with a damp cloth.

Toss a cup of powdered milk in the tub, then run the water.

Pour a teaspoon of baby oil into the bath water.

BED BUGS — Mix one ounce of corrosive sublimate (mercuric chloride) with one pint of turpentine. Mix well in a glass bottle and apply to the infected area.

BED SORES (TO PREVENT) — Bed sores occur on a patient who lies in one position, due to continued pressure on parts whose general vitality is weakened. They usually form at the lower end of the backbone. To prevent them, keep the sheet under the patient smooth, clean, and dry. Avoid pressure on any one point by changing the position frequently. When the skin is not broken, sponge the parts resting most heavily on the bed with alcohol or whiskey and water three or four times daily. Air cushions are useful. They are made to remove pressure from the lower end of the backbone.

BEDWETTING — Spray the bedwetter's pillow with wine vinegar.

Give the bedwetter three bone-meal tablets every day, after breakfast and dinner and before he goes to bed.

Have him drink four ounces of cranberry juice every day at 5:00 P.M.

At bedtime have the bedwetter eat one tablespoon of local honey.

Bedwetters should take vitamins acquired from natural sources.

Make a tea by adding ten to fifteen drops of corn silk extract to a cup of boiled water. Have the bedwetter drink this tea just before going to bed.

At night tie a towel with the knot in front around the bedwetter's loins. This encourages him to sleep on his back, which seems to lessen the urge to wet the bed.

BEEF (TO CORN) — Put six gallons of pure water in a large wash kettle and add six pounds of saltpeter. Boil. When the saltpeter is dissolved, immerse beef that has been cut into small pieces for family use. Hold it in the water on a large flesh fork or long hook. Keep it in there while you count to ten. Take it out and cool. Pack it closely and firmly in a cask or barrel. Add nine pounds of fine salt to boiling saltpeter water, then add three pounds of pure, dry sugar, one quart of your best molasses, and one pound of pearlash. Boil slowly, and skim off impurities. If the water has boiled long, while immersing beef, add a half-gallon more to replace loss from evaporation. When the pickling mixture is cold, pour it over the beef and hold the beef down by a heavy weight. Scalding of beef in saltpeter water closes the pores, prevents the juice of the meat from going into the pickle, and you have a juicy, compact, tender piece of beef, as inviting as the rump roast of a stall-fed ox, and deliciously flavored.

BEEKEEPERS — Those who keep bees do not have kidney trouble. They have clear complexions, good eyesight, and no lameness. Among those who eat honey and keep bees, there is no cancer or paralysis.

An old beekeeper says that to keep from getting stung when swarmed, you should hold your breath momentarily. The bees can't sting you because they can't get their stingers in. So they take off.

BEE STING (TO RELIEVE) — Mix some salt with water and apply.

Remove the stinger and apply a paste of soda and water.

The bee leaves a stinger along with a poison sac. If stung, attempt to remove the stinger without squeezing the poison sac. Scrape it off with a knife or fingernail.

Take a pinch of common salt, put it on the place stung and dissolve with water. Rub gently with your finger. If you feel no relief within two minutes, wet the place with aqua ammonia. Do not get ammonia in your eyes.

Use garlic oil.

BEETS — Beets practically pop right out of their skins after they're boiled if they're dipped in cold water.

BILIOUSNESS (REMEDY FOR) — If victims of this condition will exercise care, they need not panic for "anti-bilious pills." Bile doesn't belong in the stomach but gets there as a consequence of improper food, too much of the oily foods such as butter, pork, lard, etc. Bile is nature's purifying medicine, passing from the liver to the bowels. When the liver is overworked or too much greasy food is present, digestion is impaired and the whole system gets out of order. To avoid biliousness, fast for one or more meals. When the mouth tastes bad and the tongue is coated, too much food has been eaten. The appetite will fade, thus allowing nature to take over, the accumulated food to pass off, and the system to be relieved. In nine cases out of ten, this fasting will end the difficulty, save a fit of sickness, and cheat the doctor. Any quack medicine that will do as much for you as fasting would yield a fortune to the inventor. Many of them, however, increase disease rather than improve health.

BIRDS — Put pie pans up in your yard, and the birds will not eat your grass seed.

BIRTH — To ease the pain of childbirth, fix some immortelle (a member of the milkweed family) tea.

Taking calcium at the onset of labor will make delivery easier.

To ease the pain of childbirth, drink raspberry tea. Pour one pint of boiling water over one ounce of raspberry leaves, cover, and let steep for thirty minutes. Strain. Drink as hot as possible as the time for delivery approaches.

Will the baby be a boy or a girl? If it is conceived during a full moon, there is a 97 percent chance that it will be a boy. If it is conceived during a period of no moon, there is a 97 percent chance it will be a girl.

To increase milk supply, breast-feeding mothers should take brewer's yeast.

BITES AND STINGS (INSECT) — Did you know that if you take two tablespoons of brewer's yeast with your daily diet, it will keep the mosquitoes from biting you?

BLACKBERRY PICKERS — To ward off ticks and chiggers, mix one tablespoon of sulphur with a little molasses and take one hour before going out to pick the berries.

BLACKHEADS — Place hot towels on your face and neck, followed by a washing with mild soap. Then apply cold cloths and pat dry.

BLADDER (INFECTION) — Avoid tub baths in favor of showers if bladder infection (cystitis) keeps recurring.

Mix one tablespoon of apple cider vinegar and one tablespoon of honey with eight ounces of water. Take three times daily.

Eat one-half of a raw potato daily.

BLEEDING (HOW TO STOP) — A weak solution of cider vinegar applied to cuts and wounds should stop bleeding.

If you bruise or bleed easily, try eating the velvety white linings of oranges or lemons. Other sources are plums, apricots, blackberries, and green peppers, especially peppers, if you eat those velvety white inner fibers. Don't forget to eat the seeds.

BLIGHT (FRUIT TREES) — Mix one-half pound of tobacco, one-half pound of sulphur, and one peck of unslacked lime with four gallons of water. Put on or in trees.

Wind straw rope around the trunk to the first limb. Be sure this completely covers the tree to the first limb.

BLINDNESS (NIGHT) — Eat two carrots, either raw or cooked, every day.

When they are in season, eat blueberries.

Eat watercress.

B

BLOOD (CLOTS) — Crossing your legs is the most common cause of blood clots.

If you must sit for long periods of time, get up and walk around at least once every two hours.

BLOOD (FORTIFIERS) — After every meal eat four tablespoons of raw sauerkraut.

Eat peaches to wash away toxins.

Drink fresh carrot juice.

Every two hours, from morning until two hours before bedtime, take two tablespoons of a mixture of two tablespoons of lemon juice and one tablespoon of honey in a cup of warm water. For one day eat this and nothing else. (Note: Consult your doctor before going on this fast.)

Eat raw pumpkin pulp or squash.

Eat raw garlic to thin and fortify the blood.

BLOOD (LOW, REMEDY) — Eat chickweed for iron-poor blood.

Violet leaves in a tea and the roots of yellow dock are both good blood purifiers.

To remedy low blood, make a tea out of the leaves and blooms of red clover.

BLOOD PRESSURE (HIGH) — Eat two apples every day.

Watch fish in an aquarium to help you relax.

If protein intake is the cause of the high blood pressure, mix two tablespoons of apple cider vinegar with a glass of water and drink the mixture. After thirty minutes, the pressure should drop.

Eat a cucumber a day or drink one-half cup of cucumber juice.

Boil unpeeled potatoes in a pan of water for fifteen minutes. Let the water cool, then drink two cups of it per day.

Laugh more.

Eat raw garlic or take three garlic capsules a day.

This daily breathing exercise may help: Lie flat on your back on the floor, breathe in slowly (to the count of ten), hold for two seconds, then breathe out slowly (to the count of ten). Do this three to five minutes each day.

Black licorice or licorice extracts should be avoided.

Avoid all forms of tobacco.

Make a conscious effort to breathe when straining. Holding your breath during strain causes blood pressure to skyrocket.

Pets can also help to reduce high blood pressure.

BLOOD PRESSURE (LOW) — Coffee can help raise blood pressure. You should drink two cups of coffee in the morning, then avoid the beverage for the rest of the day.

BLOSSOMS (FLOWER) — To make blossoms brighter, spray with a mixture of one part water and one part brandy. A mist spray is best.

BLUES — For the "lying-around" blues, take yellowroot. Yellowroot is one of the first herbs to flower in March. When it is cut and broken, yellowroot produces a very bitter, orange-red juice. Take some of this juice. It will make you want to get up and go.

BODY WEAKNESS AND EXHAUSTION — This condition is not improved by rest.

Avoid acid-reacting foods such as potatoes, white bread, fried or greasy foods, and cakes and pastries.

Get your bowels regulated.

Do no work for sixty days.

Some suggest taking ragweed tea.

BOILS — Apply poultices of crushed raw potatoes or mashed roasted onions.

Apply poultices made of either warm milk and flour or bread crumbs and honey.

Apply vitamin-E oil on the boil and bandage. Do this three times a day.

Apply ointments of vitamins A, D, and E.

Get plenty of vitamins A and C and the minerals zinc and iron in your diet.

Slowly heat one cup of milk. As the milk approaches boiling, add three teaspoons of salt. Remove from the heat and add flour to thicken the mixture and make a poultice. Apply to the boil.

Peel off the skin of a hard-boiled egg. Wet the membrane and apply it to the boil.

Lay fresh slices of pumpkin on the boil.

Apply a poultice made of garlic (raw or cooked) to the boil.

Heat a lemon and then slice it in half. Apply the inside of one-half of the lemon to the boil for an hour.

You can also roast a fresh fig and place one-half of it on the boil for a couple of hours. Then replace it with the other half.

When the boil breaks, add two tablespoons of lemon juice to a cup of boiled water. Let it cool and then thoroughly clean the area.

BONE (PROTECTION) — Take bone-meal, calcium, or dolomite tablets.

BONE MEAL (AS PROTECTION FROM POTATO BUGS) — Before planting potatoes, roll them in bone meal so that a little adheres to the damp cuts. You will have little trouble with potato bugs.

BORERS (TO PROTECT TREES FROM) — An Ohio farmer washes his apple trees every spring and fall with a strong lye that is sure to kill borers. He claims that he has not lost a tree since beginning this practice although he had previously lost several.

BOTTLES (CLEAN) — Crush eggshells into small pieces and place the pieces inside a bottle. Fill the bottle one-quarter full with water and shake well. The inside of the bottle will sparkle.

BOWELS (TO REGULATE) — Eat a handful of clean wheat bran once or twice a day. Drink plenty of water after eating the bran.

Hot, wet cloths placed on the abdomen should relieve irritation of the bowels.

BOX (MEASURES) — Farmers and market gardeners find a series of box measures very useful, and they can be made by anyone who understands the two-foot rule and can handle a saw and a hammer. A box sixteen by sixteen and one-eighth inches square and eight inches deep will hold a bushel, or 2150.4 cubic inches, each inch in depth holding one gallon.

BRAIN (STIMULANT) — The best thing for a man to do when he feels weak is to go to bed and sleep for as long as he can. This is the only recuperation for brain power, the only real recuperation for brain force. During sleep, the brain is in a state of rest, in a condition to receive particles of nutriment, which replace those that have been used by previous labor, since even thinking burns up solid particles.

BRAN — Try eating three teaspoons of unprocessed bran with each meal. It is good for your bowels, helping to prevent constipation. It has been said that people who eat plenty of fibrous, unrefined foods seldom, if ever, get cancer of the colon.

BRASS AND COPPER (TO CLEAN) — Use coal ashes. Coal ashes are also good for scouring knives and forks.

A solution of salt and vinegar will quickly clean unlacquered brassware or copper.

BREAD (HINTS) — To freshen stale bread, dip the loaf, wrapped in a clean cloth, into boiling water; let it remain there for half a minute, then take off the cloth and bake the loaf for ten minutes in a slow oven.

Did you know that day-old bread makes better toast than fresh bread?

A good way to prepare stale bread is to store in a cool place the yolks of eggs left over after using the egg whites in cakes. The next morning beat the yolks well and dip slices of the stale bread into them. Fry the dipped bread until it is brown.

Rolls and muffins that have hardened to the "can't-be-et" stage are easily freshened. Sprinkle them with water, place them in a brown paper bag, and warm them in a hot oven for a few moments.

BREASTS (PROBLEMS) — Do not eat foods containing methylxanthines (coffee, tea, colas, and chocolate). These can trigger the development of cysts in sensitive women.

Take vitamin E three times daily.

BREATH (BAD) — Drink plenty of water and use a humidifier to help relieve bad breath caused by dryness.

Gargle with this mixture: Bring two cups of water to a boil. Place several coarsely chopped sprigs of parsley, two or three whole cloves or one-quarter teaspoon of ground cloves, one teaspoon of powdered myrrh, and one teaspoon of powdered goldenseal into the boiling water. Strain and use the clear liquid as a mouthwash or gargle.

Lick the back of your hand, wait two minutes, then smell the area you licked. This test will tell you whether you have bad breath or not.

BRONCHITIS — Mix the juice of two lemons, which have been warmed in an oven to dry the skins, four ounces of your best honey, and two teaspoons of the very finest Florence oil. Put the mixture in an earthen jar and keep the jar covered. Swallow a spoonful when you feel a fit coming on. (This treatment can also be effective for asthma.)

For a cold complicated by bronchitis, rub your chest with castor oil and turpentine.

To treat bronchitis, put two drops of creosote into a bottle that will hold a pint or so. Pour in a little more than half a pint of clear water and shake well. Always shake before using. Gargle a mouthful of this mixture for a little while, then swallow it. Repeat every two hours, more or less, so as to use up the liquid within twenty-four hours. For each subsequent twenty-four hours, use three drops of creosote in three to four gills of water. This three drops a day may be continued as long as any bronchitis appears. Two to four days is usually enough, though the treatment may be continued indefinitely without harm.

Inhale brandy fumes twice a day.

Eat onions, raw or cooked.

Avoid quick or drastic changes in heat or cold or vigorous exercises.

Vitamin A may help.

Avoid strong odors and emotional stress.

For some, drinking two cups of coffee in the morning helps (drink no coffee for the rest of the day).

Mix one tablespoon of apple-cider vinegar and one tablespoon of honey with eight ounces of water. Take three times daily.

BROOM (TIPS) — A new broom should be soaked in hot, heavily salted water to give it a longer life.

Put a rubber tip on the handle of your broom.

To keep the broom from wearing out quickly, dip the ends of the bristles into a shallow pan of thinned shellac.

BRUISES — Apply cornstarch.

Apply some ground white onions to the bruise. Leave them on for at least eight hours.

Eat more oranges, lemons, and green peppers.

Drink one quart of orange juice a day.

BRUSHES (PAINT) — Soak neglected paintbrushes in hot vinegar to clean and make them as pliable as new ones.

BUCKEYE — Carry a buckeye in your pocket to ward off rheumatism.

BUNION (CURE) — Apply iodine, freely, twice a day with a feather. For cure of corns or chilblains, the same treatment is recommended.

Apply a plaster consisting of ten drops of iodine mixed with one-half teaspoon of lard. Bandage the foot twice a day. This treatment also works for corns.

BURNS — Put the burned part of body in cold water as soon as possible.

When wheat is green and in head, cut a handful off about one foot below the head (include head). Do not wash. Cut into pieces small enough to fit into a skillet or pan. Fry in hog lard until the pieces are really brown but don't burn them. When the wheat is done, take it out and throw it away. Strain the lard through a clean white cloth. Store the strained lard in a covered jar. It will keep a long time. Use as needed on burns.

The following treatments are for all but the most serious kinds of burns in which large areas of skin are destroyed:

Apply cool water and/or apply the juice of the aloe vera plant.

Apply vitamin-E powder, vitamin-E oil, or vitamin-E cream.

Wash the burned area with cold water and smother with honey. Wrap with a white towel.

Bandage with a cloth soaked in white vinegar. Apply white vinegar to the cloth to keep it from drying out.

Smear the burn with the white of an egg.

Apply scraped raw potato to the burn and bandage.

Apply yogurt three times daily.

Soak the burned area in vitamin-C solution.

Spray the burned area with the same solution of vitamin C.

Pour the white of an egg over a burn or scald. It is softer than collodion, and, being convenient, the egg white can be applied immediately. It is more cooling than sweet oil and cotton, which was formerly thought to be the surest application to ease the pain of a burn.

Contact with air gives discomfort to the wound, and anything that keeps air out and prevents inflammation is an appropriate thing to apply.

Sprinkle on a few grains of white sugar if you should accidentally burn your tongue. It should relieve the pain.

Apply pumpkin-seed oil to the burn.

Apply fresh pumpkin pulp or a slice of raw onion to the burn. Leave on for fifteen minutes, remove for five minutes, then replace with a fresh piece for another fifteen minutes.

Apply garlic oil to the burn.

Uncooked chicken fat will soothe a burn.

Place a smooth piece of charcoal on the burn for an hour.

Use a poultice of raw sauerkraut.

If you happen to burn yourself outdoors, pack mud on the burned area.

Spread apple butter on the burn.

Pour apple cider vinegar on the burned area.

Put the petals of some large white lilies in a jar, cover with olive oil, close the jar, and keep it for the times when the treatment is needed. When a burn occurs, take a leaf or two from the jar and place them on the burn. Replace the leaves when the oil dries. This potion will keep for years.

Mix equal parts of lime water with either olive oil or linseed oil. Apply as needed to burns.

Rinse your mouth with cold water if you burn your tongue. Apply a few drops of vanilla extract.

BURSITIS — Apply cod-liver oil and massage the affected area.

Eat a high-fiber diet.

Mix one tablespoon of apple-cider vinegar with eight ounces of water. Take three times daily.

Exercise in moderation.

Avoid red meats, fried foods, sugar, grease, and white-flour products.

Place warm castor-oil packs over affected areas.

Apply Epsom-salt packs.

Do not drink carbonated beverages or alcoholic drinks.

BUTTER (TO COLOR) — Deep yellow carrots give the most natural color and best flavor to butter when you are coloring it. Take two large carrots, clean them, then scrape off the yellow part, leaving the white pith. Soak the yellow part in boiling milk for about ten minutes. Strain the mixture while it is still hot into the cream to be used for butter.

BUTTERMILK — Buttermilk is good, especially for a patient with a fever, as an article of diet. A cup of fresh buttermilk every day is a cure for liver complaints.

BUTTERMILK (AS A CLEANSER) — Soak a sponge in buttermilk for five hours, squeeze it out, and wash it in cold water. Add a little lemon juice to the rinse water.

BUTTONS (TO REMOVE) — In removing buttons from clothing, you won't snip the fabric if you slide a comb under the button and cut the thread carefully with a razor blade.

Back Pain Zapper

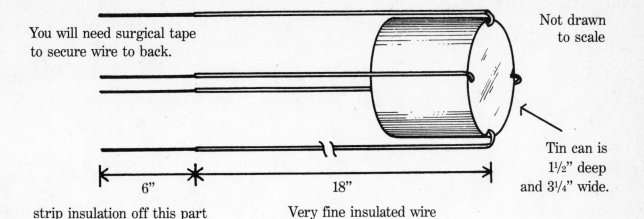

You will need surgical tape to secure wire to back.

Not drawn to scale

Tin can is 1½" deep and 3¼" wide.

6"

18"

strip insulation off this part

Very fine insulated wire

1. Prepare the following items: one tin can one and one-half inches deep and three and one-quarter inches wide and four twenty-four-inch pieces of very fine insulated copper wire.

2. Strip off six inches of the insulation on one end of each wire .

3. On the other end of each wire, strip off one-quarter inch of the insulation.

4. Close to the end of the tin can, bore four holes the size of the copper wire.

5. Place one one-quarter-inch piece of copper wire through each hole in the tin can and solder.

6. Curl each six-inch end of copper wire close to the spot that hurts on your back.

7. Secure the curled copper wire to your back with surgical tape.

8. Hold the tin can in one hand. Then take a twelve-inch wooden ruler with the other hand and rub it across the top of the tin can for two minutes. Rest for five minutes and repeat.

9. Do this five times a day for three days.

10. Between treatments, place hot castor-oil packs on the back every other day. On the alternate day, place hot apple-cider-vinegar packs on the back.

11. Also, after each treatment, lie on your back while taking in a deep breath and raising the feet and head off the floor. While the feet and head are off the floor, count to twenty. Exhale and lower the feet and head to the floor. Repeat this ten times after each treatment. Do not exhale while counting to twenty.

*Cooks—Send Dick your
ten best baking secrets.*

1. _____

2. _____

3. _____

4. _____

5. _____

6. _____

7. _____

8. _____

9. _____

10. _____

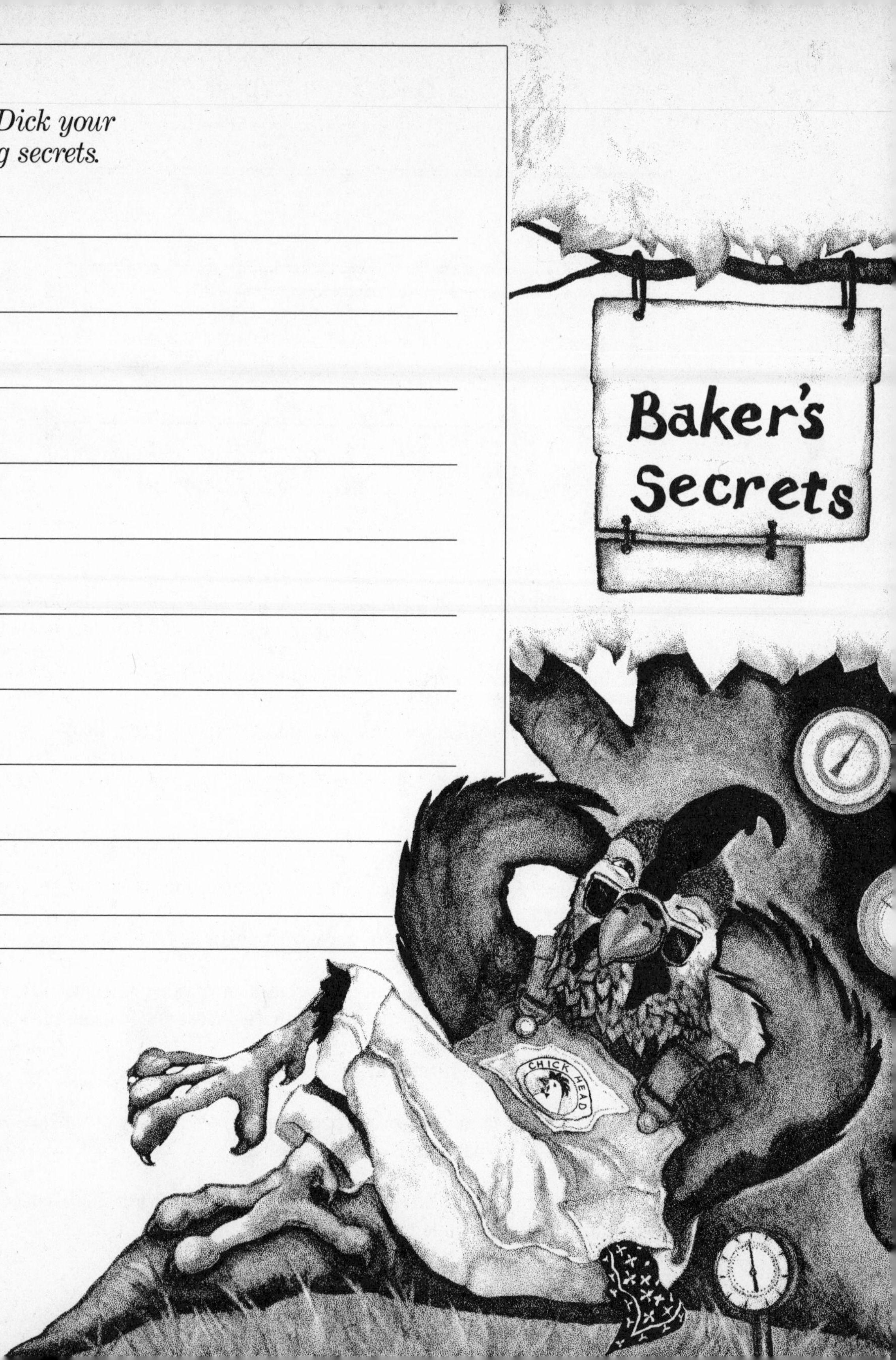

Baker's
Secrets

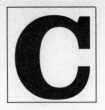

CABBAGE (GRUBS) — To destroy white grubs at the root of cabbages, loosen the earth close to the root with a hoe. Make a solution of one quart of soft soap to twelve quarts of soft water and pour the mixture about the root in close contact with the plant. One-fourth of a pint of this solution applied to a plant two or three times during the season is sufficient. Weaker suds poured on top should destroy the green worm.

CABBAGE (MADE DIGESTIBLE) — First slice the cabbage. Then put it in boiling water with a pinch of soda and some salt and boil fifteen minutes.

CABBAGE (RED) — Red cabbage will keep its color if you add some lemon juice or vinegar to the cooking water.

CAKE — Your beautiful cake won't stick to the pan if you'll grease the one in which it's to be baked with a fat containing no salt. Then lightly dust flour over the fat.

To tell if the cake is done, pierce it with an ordinary toothpick. If it comes out clean, your cake is ready.

Fill cake pans only half full with batter for the best results. Running over the rims of the pan is wasteful.

To frost a cake neatly, cover the edge of the cake plate with triangles of waxed paper. Place the cake on these and frost it. Then gently draw the papers away, leaving the plate clean. For an expert frosting job, spread the frosting first from the top edge down over the sides. Pile the remaining frosting on the top and spread lightly to the edges.

If you want to make wonderful looking cakes, it pays to frost them first with a thin layer of icing. This will hold down crumbs and give an even base coat. After this first coat is set, the final frosting goes on easily and will look extra glamorous.

CALAMUS (ROOT) — Chew and swallow the juice of *Acorus calamus* instead of Rolaids or Tums. It tastes bad, but if you eat too much or have a sour, burning stomach, it makes you feel better.

CALCIUM — Nothing is 100 percent for sure, and I don't guarantee anything, but if I were you, I would start increasing your calcium intake now. You will find it the best way to improve the odds against developing osteoporosis (thinning of the bones).

Discuss this with your family doctor and hope that he or she understands the effects of dietary habits on bone development and density.

C

Just how much calcium is enough? I would say one thousand milligrams a day. An eight-ounce glass of milk (whole, low-fat, or skim) contains 290 milligrams—almost a third of the RDA (Recommended Daily Allowance). For anyone who is lactose intolerant, an equivalent amount of calcium is available in a cup of yogurt. Other sources include oysters, salmon, and sardines (eaten with bones).

CALCIUM (DEPOSITS) — Place castor-oil packs over the deposits. This will help stimulate the body to reabsorb the calcium. Drink potato juice to increase your body's alkaline content.

CAMOMILE — Camomile is rich in calcium and potassium. It will help to heal nervous disorders, sleeplessness, menstrual problems, and stomachaches.

CAMPERS (TIPS) — Along with dry matches, pack lint from the clothes dryer into a small plastic pill bottle. It ignites quickly and can make tinder for several fires. It's light in weight and takes no space.

When camping without any refrigeration, coat your eggs with shortening. This will help preserve them by sealing out air.

During cold-weather camping, wear wool clothing. If you get wet accidentally, wool will continue to keep you warm while other fibers won't.

If your boots get wet while you are camping, pull some rocks from the campfire and put your boots upside down over them.

CANARIES (CARE OF) — Don't put canaries in a painted cage. They pick the wires and will be poisoned. Brass wire cages are more cheerful than wood and can be easily cleaned.

Give the birds fresh seed, pure water, both for drinking and bathing, cuttlefish, and, in season, fresh lettuce and chickweed. Cake is harmful.

To keep the cage clean, a piece of brown paper covering the bottom is helpful, as it can be replaced every morning. Never use newspaper because the birds pick the ink. After the birds bathe, take the bath out of the cage. If it stands all day, it becomes impure, and the birds are better bathers if the dish is placed in the cage at a regular time. Keep the perches clean, which you can do easily by rubbing them with sandpaper. Give the birds fresh sand every day.

Supply fresh air and plenty of sunshine. Guard against drafts and extreme heat. The noon sunshine should not fall directly on the cage.

Baker's sponge cake dipped in sherry is strongly recommended for sick canaries that have been moulting. The bird will no doubt eat sparingly of it, but the remedy is good. It has been known to restore the voice and health of canaries that have been shedding for eighteen months or two years. Birds often continue moulting from weakness, and a short time of feeding them on cake and sherry, in connection with their seed, soon produces an improvement. I would also advise not giving a bird in this condition any greens or apples to eat.

Canaries with asthma can get relief and sometimes be cured by eating a pap made of baker's bread boiled in sweet milk. In very bad cases, remove the sick bird's seed for a few days and let it feed entirely on this pap.

The following treatment restores a sick and silent bird: Leave off its seed entirely. Make a paste of sweet milk and bread crumbs. Throw the crumbs into the milk while it is boiling and stir until the mixture is smooth. Add a pinch of cayenne pepper, varying the mix occasionally with finely minced clove or garlic. Dissolve in drinking water a little black currant jelly, a bit of fig, or half a potash lozenge. It may take a long time to cure the bird, and if the trouble arises from hardness of the tongue, paint the tongue daily with strong borax water. If the bird sneezes, put a little olive oil up its nostrils. The sick bird should have plenty of warm water to bathe in and celery, sweet apple, or lettuce. Do not hang the bird close to the window because the cold is too severe for a sick bird even in a warm room. The paste must be fresh daily.

CANCER — Drinking two or three glasses of skim milk each day may help prevent colorectal cancer. Do not take vitamin-D supplements while drinking a lot of vitamin-D fortified milk.

Avoid exposing your skin and eyes to the ultraviolet rays of the sun. Wear protective sunglasses, hats, or visors when you are in the sun.

Increase your intake of fruits and vegetables to reduce your risks of certain types of stomach cancer.

Garlic and onions are also being studied as possible means of slowing the progress of cancer.

Eggs, fried foods, and coffee should be avoided.

A high-fiber diet and plenty of exercise can help people who have a desk job reduce their risk of colon cancer. Those with desk jobs have a higher risk of this particular kind of cancer.

Calcium supplements may also reduce the risk of colon cancer.

Limit your intake of pickled and cured foods.

CANCER (LUNG) — Inhale apple-brandy fumes.

Apply warm castor-oil packs.

CANCER (OLD-TIME CURE) — Take some red clover blossoms and make a tea out of them. Old-timers claimed it would cure cancer of the stomach and also surface cancer. Drink this tea three times a day.

If you have a tendency toward cancer, eat a few almonds each day.

CANCER (SKIN) — Massage the gel of an aloe plant on the spots.

CANDLE — Don't risk wobbly candles! Melt some paraffin, pour it into the socket, and put the candle in while it's hot.

Chill candles in the refrigerator for twenty-four hours before using them on the table. They will burn evenly and will not drip.

CANKER AND COLD SORES — These sores act as an early warning signal that a person has digestive problems or bowel movement difficulties, which contribute to excess acidity in the system. Here are some things a person can do:

Eat more alkaline-reacting foods, such as raw and cooked leafy greens and citrus fruits.

Avoid foods containing fats and starches and those which are acid producing.

Massage the back and spine with olive oil.

Rinse out the mouth with Lavoris.

Avoid carbonated drinks, fried foods, and cake and pastries.

Hold ice cubes directly against an erupted sore for forty-five minutes, four times a day, for two days.

Apply myrrh in an alcohol solution with a cotton swab. Just touch the center of the sore.

Eat yogurt.

Take lysine.

Take two acidophilus capsules thirty minutes before each meal.

Apply liquid vitamin E to the sore.

Take four drops of vitamin E three times a day.

CARPET (TO RESTORE FADED) — Dip the carpet in strong salt and water. (Blue factory cotton or silk handkerchiefs will not fade if dipped in salt water while they are new.)

CARROTS — Cut carrots and other long vegetables lengthwise when you cook them. This way less of the nutritional value will be lost during cooking.

CASTOR OIL (HOT PACKS) — Heat the oil, and place three or four layers of flannel in it. Wring out and apply. Place a dry heating pad over the pack. When treatment is done, bathe with a weak baking-soda solution. This will cleanse the body of acidity and promote natural secretions. Most packs should be applied over the right abdomen for five days, for one and one-half hours each time.

CATARACTS (TO HELP PREVENT) — Eat a well-balanced diet.

Apply potato poultices to the eyes and back.

CATNIP — Catnip (*Nepeta cataria*) tea is good for headaches and pacifying babies. It'll do away with the hives, and if your stomach doesn't digest its food, this tea will help start the digestive process.

CATS' PROBLEMS — For injuries, clean the wound and apply vitamin E.

For sores, crush one-half zinc tablet and mix with Vaseline. Apply to the sore two times a day. Give the other one-half tablet to the cat. Do this each day for a week.

Give high-potency yeast tablets every day for fifteen days to cats with skin and fur problems.

Try desiccated liver for cats with infections of the reproductive organs.

For urinary problems, try this diet for your cat: chicken, potatoes, liver, red beets, cabbage, corn, carrots, and fish. Use no salt in the preparation of these foods for the cat. Add a little tomato juice and water to each meal.

Sprinkle one-quarter teaspoon of brewer's yeast over the food of a cat with fleas. (This treatment is also good for dermatitis.) Ten milligrams of thiamine daily may also help with fleas and ticks. Another flea treatment is to add one teaspoon of pennyroyal oil to four tablespoons of spring water. Rub the mixture on your cat once a month.

If your cat has diarrhea, give it four viable yogurt culture tablets each day. (You must keep these tablets in the refrigerator.) After five days, add two desiccated-liver capsules each day. Crush the tablets and mix them with the cat's food.

For a cat that is nervous, vomiting, and licking constantly, try dolomite tablets and one-quarter teaspoon of crushed bone meal with its food.

Avoid feeding your cat fatty fish, veal, pork, starches, such as potatoes, spinach greens, and milk (for adult cats, if it often causes diarrhea).

To keep cats off of your car, put moth balls in a piece of cloth and put it on the hood of your car or sprinkle the hood and top of the car with black pepper.

CAULIFLOWER — Don't waste cauliflower stalks. Eat them. They're delicious cooked. Serve them with a white or Hollandaise sauce.

CAYENNE PEPPER — This herb is important in many kinds of first aid. As a seasoning, it helps to bring out the flavor in food.

CELERY — Why waste celery tops? Cut them up and use them to flavor meats, stews, soups, roasts, and stuffings.

CEREAL — Use cereal to stretch meats. Add crushed cereal flakes to a meat loaf. Or toss cereal flakes with melted margarine and grated cheese for a casserole topping.

CHAIR (CANE-BOTTOMED, TO RESTORE) — Turn the chair bottom upward and, with hot water and a sponge, wash the cane work so that it is well-soaked. If the caning is dirty, use soap. Let the chair dry in the air, and it will be as tight and firm as new, provided none of the canes is broken.

C

CHAMOIS (STIFF) — Soak stiff chamois in warm water with a spoonful of olive oil.

CHEESE — Periodically grate all the ends and scraps of hard cheese left in the refrigerator. Different kinds can be mixed and stored in a jar. You'll be glad you did this when a recipe calls for a handful of grated cheese and it's ready instantly.

CHEST (CONGESTION) — Fix some eneldo (related to dill) tea.

CHICKEN POX — Cook some oatmeal and put it in a cloth bag. Float this in a tub of warm water, and swish it around until the water becomes silky. Do not break the bag. If you do, you will have a slimy mess! Let the child with chicken pox play in this water. Leave the pouch of oatmeal in the tub. Be sure the water goes all over the scabs, but don't allow the child to get chilled. Do this two times a day.

For additional relief from chicken pox, boil some willow leaves and pour the "tea" into bath water. This is very soothing, and many say there will be no itching if you do this.

Be sure the patient maintains good bowel movements.

Do not let the patient catch cold.

Avoid feeding the patient acid-forming foods.

Apply honey or vitamin-E oil to the sores.

CHICKENS — Finely chopped onions given two or three times a week will help prevent sickness in chickens.

To cure thickening of the membrane of the tongue in chickens, take a lump of butter and mix some Scotch snuff with it. Put two or three large pills of this down the chicken's throat. Keep the chicken out of cold, damp places, and it will recover.

The left leg of the chicken is more tender than the right. A chicken usually sleeps on the right leg, which then develops tougher tendons and muscles.

Directions for raising chickens:
1) Avoid damp floors in the chicken house.
2) Provide lots of sunshine.
3) Provide one rooster for every twelve hens.
4) Scatter their food so they can't eat too fast.
5) Keep the hen house clean and ventilated.
6) Do not overcrowd the hen house.
7) An unhappy hen will not produce good eggs.
8) Whitewash roosts and the bottom of laying nests once a month.
9) No chickens should be over four years old.
10) Keep the best chickens for breeding purposes.

11) To keep the hens laying in cold weather, give them some warm milk with a dash of pepper in it.

12) Boiled vegetables, mixed with milk and barley, will speed up the fattening process.

13) Feed corn to setting chickens.

14) Feed young chicks cracked corn. When chicks are two or three weeks old, feed them whole grains of corn. This will prevent or cure the gapes, the rodworms that get in their throats.

15) Put some old nails in their drinking water.

Small amounts of pulverized charcoal added to chicken (or turkey) feed will make the birds gain weight faster.

CHIGGER (BITES) — Gather a few bunches of pennyroyal and boil them into a strong tea. Put this tea on the bites. It will ease the itching.

CHILD TRAINING AND PROBLEMS WITH BEHAVIOR — Massage the back (not the spine) with olive oil by moving up and down each side of the spine. Rub in small circles on both sides of the spine. Use a clockwise motion on the right side and a counterclockwise motion on the left. Work from top to bottom.

Talk to the child about his or her dreams and imagination and about nature and God.

Never give your child something because he or she cries for it.

Never allow your children to do something that you have formerly forbidden.

Teach your children that the only way to appear good is to be good.

Never allow lying.

Teach children self-denial, not self-indulgence.

From the earliest infancy, inculcate the necessity of instant obedience.

Let your children always understand that you mean what you say.

Never promise children anything unless you are sure that you can give it to them.

If you tell a child to do something, show him how to do it and see that it is done.

Never punish your child in anger, but you should always punish him or her for willfully disobeying you.

Never let your children know that they make you lose your self-command.

A present punishment is much more effectual than the promise of a greater punishment should the fault arise again.

CHILLS — Place a scraped Irish potato in a cloth and put it on the hollow of the throat.

CHIMNEY (CLEAN) — Chimneys need to be cleaned after three or four cords of wood have been burned and more often if the wood is soft and green.

Place a piece of zinc on the live coals in the fireplace or stove. The zinc will produce a vapor, and this in turn will carry off the soot by chemical decomposition.

CHIMNEY LAMP (HOW TO CLEAN) — Wash in soda and water.

CHINA — When packing china for storage or moving, don't use newspaper. The ink can rub off onto the dishes, and they will have to be rewashed.

Mix flour with the white of an egg to the consistency of a paste and use as a cement for mending broken china.

CHIPS (KEEP FRESH) — Use a clothespin to close bags of chips after folding over the tops.

CHOLESTEROL (HIGH) — Soft yellowish patches around the eyes, particularly on the eyelids, may signal an elevated cholesterol level.

Mix one tablespoon of apple-cider vinegar and one tablespoon of local honey with one cup of water. Take three times daily. If you are a diabetic, leave off the honey.

Eat one-half of a raw potato (small to medium) daily.

Eat one-half cup of fresh strawberries daily.

Eat a high-fiber diet.

When you eat grapefruit, be sure to eat part of the inner white peel.

Do not eat anything that has been treated with daminozide.

CIGARETTE (SMOKE) — Install window fans or buy an air-purifying system. Saucers of vinegar will dissipate cigarette smoke, as will candles.

CIRCULATION (PROBLEMS) — Try the hot and cold treatment. Place the arm, leg, or whatever part suffers from poor circulation in cold water for ten seconds, then in warm water for about twenty seconds, alternating back and forth in that manner for a period of ten minutes. Do this three or four times a day. You have nothing to lose.

Drink one-eighth of a teaspoon of cayenne pepper in a cup of water daily.

Soak your feet in two quarts of warm water to which a cup of fresh minced ginger has been added.

Take two lecithin capsules and one four-hundred-I.U. vitamin-E capsule every day.

CIRRHOSIS — Eat a high-fiber diet.

Apply castor-oil packs over the liver area.

Take one teaspoonful of olive oil daily.

CLEAN (HOUSE) — Mix equal parts of distilled white vinegar and water. It's a good all-purpose cleaner for walls, counter tops, glass, and bathrooms.

Lemon juice is a good grease cutter. For furniture polish, mix two parts olive oil or vegetable oil with one part lemon juice.

Mix borax with hot water to wipe away mold and mildew and as a disinfectant.

CLEANSING CREAM — Mix Crisco shortening, olive oil, glycerin, lanolin, and castor oil in the blender and use as a cleansing cream.

CLOCK (SOUNDPROOF) — Cover a clock with a large glass jar or bowl if the ticking disturbs you.

CLOTHESPINS — Wash clothespins in a saltwater solution before using them. They will last longer. They will not freeze on the clothes if you need to hang something out in the winter months.

CLOTHING (CARE OF) — Make a small slit in the sewn end of pillow cases to make your own garment bags.

Store lace in waxed paper to keep it looking nice and lasting longer.

Place a bowl of water with a sponge in it in the closet to make your own humidified closet. Water must be added periodically to replace the water that evaporates.

Keep a sixty-watt electric light bulb burning in your closet all the time to keep out dampness.

Store white articles in a box with a small piece of yellow soap or black tissue paper to keep them from yellowing.

If you pull old laundered socks over shoes not in use or packed for travel, they will look like new and remain separate from other packed items.

A piece of soap keeps a suitcase or bag of stored clothes smelling fresh.

If you want to wash your clothes in sea water, mix some soda with it first.

Wear rubber gloves when washing pantyhose and delicate knits. A split in your fingernail can cause runs and snags.

Rub just enough hand lotion onto your hands to moisten them. Rub it in well. Then rub the palms of your hands over pantyhose or your slip. This will take care of static cling. In the absence of hand lotion, sprinkle garments with water.

To prevent your nylon pantyhose from getting holes in the toes, rub the toe section with paraffin after each washing.

Heat a panful of clean round pebbles in the oven, pour them in your boots, and rattle them around. The moisture will be dispelled by the heat. Test for heat sensitivity by first holding a hot pebble in one spot for a few seconds.

COAT (FUR) — When your fur coat has been soaked in rain or snow, dry it in a well-ventilated room. Never dry it near heat. Brush the coat before drying it.

COCKROACHES — Cut off some cucumber peelings and place them where the roaches are each night.

Sprinkle plenty of powdered borax where roaches are seen. Be sure to renew the borax occasionally. It won't take long before no roaches will be seen. This is a very safe exterminator.

COCONUT — Dry coconut softens quickly when steamed over boiling water.

If shredded coconut gets dry, make it extra delicious by toasting it. Sprinkle it on a baking sheet and heat in a moderate oven, shaking occasionally to brown evenly.

It's easy to make lovely tinted coconut. Just fill glass half full of shredded coconut. Sprinkle in a few drops of diluted coloring. Cover the jar and shake.

COFFEE — Drink it straight; never use milk or cream in it.

COLDS — Lemon juice with sugar used freely as long as a cold remains provides some relief.

For a cough due to a cold, mix some honey with cooked onions for cough syrup.

You'll be free of colds all winter if you catch a falling leaf in your hand in autumn. Oh, how easy it sounds! But just try to catch one.

At the first sign of cold, start drinking one quart of orange juice a day. Take garlic capsules. Chew vitamin-C tablets for sore throat.

Drink yarrow or horsemint tea.

Eat a high-fiber diet.

Drink plenty of water daily.

Avoid sweets, starches, and meats.

Eat leafy green and raw vegetables.

Eat citrus fruits and drink their juices.

Eat carrots, celery, and parsley for noon meals.

Eat lettuce, celery, and kale (good blood purifiers).

Avoid fried foods and meat fats.

Sweeten with honey.

Drink the juice from steamed onions.

Apply Epsom-salt packs to the abdomen and the base of the spine.

As a digestive aid, mix one-half teaspoon baking soda with a cup of water and drink.

If you are stopped up, pour some whiskey over boiling water and breathe the fumes.

Get plenty of rest.

Spend more time outdoors.

Avoid night air and cold air.

Be sure that you have proper bowel movements.

Mix one tablespoon of cider vinegar and one tablespoon of honey with eight ounces of water. Take three times daily. If you can't take the honey, take the vinegar.

Place a paper sack over your head and breathe in and out twenty to thirty times. Do this three times daily.

For a chest cold, dip flannel in boiling water, sprinkle it with turpentine, and lay the cloth on your chest as quickly as possible.

Another remedy for a chest cold is a mustard plaster. To make one, mix one tablespoon of flour and one tablespoon of mustard powder with a small amount of water. Then add the beaten white of an egg. Put this poultice on the patient and leave it on until it begins to turn the skin red or a nice pink color. Then remove it and cover the chest with a warm woolen cloth. Keep the plaster moist in waxed paper, and when the skin is white again, warm the plaster and repeat until the skin is red again. Then remove it and keep the patient's chest well covered and warm.

Eating an apple, broccoli, and/or parsley once a day can help ward off chest colds.

Another treatment for chest colds is to take five drops of cinnamon oil in a tablespoon of water four times a day.

Drinking raw sauerkraut juice once a day is also believed to help with chest colds.

If you are coming down with a cold, eat fried onions for supper and/or eat slices of raw onion just before bedtime. This will usually knock the cold out.

Eat chicken soup three times a day, at least eight ounces each time.

Peel and crush six cloves of garlic. Mix them into one-half cup of white lard. Spread this mixture on the soles of the feet and cover them with a towel. Put paper toweling under the feet to absorb grease. Apply a fresh batch of garlic and lard every four hours.

Drink plenty of unsweetened fruit juices.

Combine three teaspoons of honey and the juice of one lemon with five teaspoons of rum. Then add it to six ounces of hot water and drink before going to bed.

Place an ice cube on the bottom of both big toes. Use an Ace bandage or a piece of cloth to keep them in place. This will stimulate appropriate points that can help a cold. Do it morning, noon, and night.

At the first sign of cold, start gargling with vinegar and salt and taking a gram of vitamin C, followed by five hundred milligrams every half-hour until bedtime, then a gram every time you wake up during the night.

Taking a hot foot bath can help. Place both feet and your lower legs into a pail of hot water (up to 110 degrees Fahrenheit) for a few minutes. Heat applied to the chest wall is also a very good treatment.

To relieve a head cold, drink some tea made as follows: Take one-half ounce each of red pepper, cinnamon, and cloves and one-half pound each of ginger and bayberry bark. Grind and mix thoroughly. Store in wide-mouthed bottles corked tightly. When needed, take a teaspoon of the mixture in a bowl of boiling water. Sugar and milk can be added to improve the taste.

Another treatment for a head cold is strong lemonade with lots of sugar. This should be taken as hot as possible. After drinking the lemonade, stay in a warm bed and do not go out into the cold.

COLIC — A pinch of soda in a spoon of water is good for colic. So is ginseng tea.

A patient with colic should be relieved within a few minutes if you turn him upside down.

Break a loaf of bread in two, hot from the oven. Place half upon the lower stomach of a patient with colic and the other half on the back opposite the first half. Relief will come shortly.

If a mother is breast-feeding her baby and the child is often colicky, she should avoid milk in her diet. Chances are fifty-fifty that this will help. Breast-feeding mothers should also avoid milk products, chocolate, caffeine, alcohol, broccoli, spicy foods, beans, brussels sprouts, carbonated drinks, melons, apples, wheat-flour products, and other foods that produce gas.

A nursing mother with a colicky baby should also try sipping camomile tea.

Giving a colicky baby a few drops of garlic oil often helps. Another treatment is to give the baby one teaspoon of olive oil the first thing in the morning, then hold off the first feeding for about an hour.

During a colic spell, give the baby one or two ounces of warm water.

Lay the baby face down with a hot-water bottle under his or her stomach.

Play soothing music or rock the baby gently.

Always feed a baby in an upright position.

Burp the baby often, and give him or her smaller feedings more often during the day.

A spoonful of calcium gluconate syrup before feeding may also help colic.

Boil a cup of water with a quarter of a bay leaf in it for fifteen minutes. Give this to the baby in a bottle.

Before giving the baby water, mix ten drops of lemon juice with four ounces of water.

Massage the baby's back with olive oil.

COLITIS — Don't eat seeds, nuts, or seedy fruits, such as blackberries and strawberries. Peel and cook fruits you do eat.

Don't take laxatives, medicines, or drugs if you can help it.

You can't go entirely without food if you are dieting. Plain digestive juices are too strong for your system.

Eat good homegrown food. The food bought in stores has chemicals that could worsen your problem.

Be happy. This will require rearranging your lifestyle. You will find that you will take better care of yourself when you are happy.

Don't wear clothes that are tight-fitting around the waist and abdomen. (Tight clothes can also cause hemorrhoids.)

Don't drink soft drinks, coffee, or tea. Onions, garlic, and salt are the only seasonings that you should use.

Eat a high-fiber diet.

Eat fruits and vegetables and drink fruit juices.

Massage the spine and abdomen with olive oil.

Drink ginseng tea.

Make a poultice out of Concord grapes and apply it to the abdomen for three hours daily for five days.

Eat seafood, fish, fowl, and raw vegetables.

Avoid sweets, fats, starches, and red meat.

Vinegar must be avoided.

COLON (STOPPED UP) — Apply a castor-oil pack to the stomach and liver area for twelve hours each day and continue for five days.

Massage the stomach and spine with olive oil.

Take one-half teaspoon of olive oil every three hours for two days.

COLOR BLINDNESS — The following might help:

Eat lots of citrus fruits and green and raw vegetables.

Eat whole-wheat bread.

Do not eat potatoes, but do eat potato peelings.

Do not eat apples or bananas.

COMBS (CLEAN) — Here's an easy, no-fuss way to clean combs: Spray them with foamy bathroom cleaner. Wait a few minutes, then rinse them in hot water.

COMPLEXION — Wash your face with buttermilk once a day. Rinse with warm water, and pat dry with a soft towel.

For a good complexion, mix six ounces of peanut oil, two ounces of olive oil, two ounces of rose water, and one tablespoon of dissolved lanolin. Massage the skin with this mixture after taking a hot bath.

If you have complexion problems, your diet is very important and should consist of easily digested foods. Eat fruit and drink fruit juices. Eat carrots and squash. Eat fish and fowl. Avoid red meats, sugar, and fried foods. Eat four almonds a day. Eat a high-fiber diet.

A problem complexion will also be helped by doing lots of walking and massaging the spine with peanut oil.

CONSTIPATION — Drink hot orange juice.

Eat a high-fiber diet. The first thing I would do is to buy some bran. Bran can be mixed with juice. Mix some in your oatmeal. You can even take it in tablet form. Start out by taking one heaping tablespoon of bran a day. Increase or decrease the amount as needed. Use unprocessed bran or unprocessed bran tablets. Dieters should be sure to eat bran each day. People who have four or more bowel movements a day are helped just as much by bran as those who are constipated.

Try this combination formula: shredded wheat, brewer's yeast, wheat germ, lecithin granules, bran, safflower oil, and low-fat skim milk.

Do not take mineral oil for more than a few days because it tends to coat the entire intestinal tract and can block absorption of important vitamins.

Eat prunes; forget the prune juice.

Always eat whole-wheat bread.

Soak eight dried figs in a glass of water overnight. In the morning, drink the water, then eat the figs.

Drink the juice of one-half lemon in one cup of warm water before breakfast.

Eat a roasted Spanish onion at bedtime.

Eat raw sauerkraut and drink its juice.

Drink one-half cup of sauerkraut juice combined with one-half cup of tomato juice.

Eat garlic.

Soak your feet in cold water twice a day, fifteen minutes each time. Dry thoroughly.

Eat spinach.

Eat okra.

Before supper eat two spoons full of raisins or four prunes that have been soaked in water for three hours.

CONSUMPTION — Drink corn-silk tea or corn-silk wine.

CONVULSIONS — Drink pennyroyal tea.

COOKING (HINTS) — When cooking raw vegetables such as carrots, potatoes, etc., put a tablespoon of shortening, butter, or vegetable oil into the water as you start cooking. The vegetables come out more flavorful and tender.

Rub butter over the cut side of an onion to keep it fresh for future use.

After handling raw meat, fish, poultry, and eggs and before touching other foods, wash your hands, knives, and cutting boards in hot, soapy water. This prevents the spread of bacteria and parasites.

Cut hot bread or cake with a hot knife.

Did you know that chili powder, cayenne pepper, and paprika need to be refrigerated?

Do not keep onions and potatoes in the same place. If you do, the potatoes will sprout. Always separate them.

Do not heat a kettle of water when all you need is a cupful. This wastes energy and time.

CORKS (ENLARGING) — To enlarge corks, boil them in a covered pan.

CORN (COOKING) — You can remove corn silks much more thoroughly by using a small, stiff brush for those last remaining strands.

Don't pick at the strands of corn silk. Wipe down the cob, from tip to base, with a damp paper towel.

To save some time, use a nylon hair net when you have finished husking an ear of corn to rub up and down the ear. It will remove all the silk that's stuck between the rows.

CORN (EARWORM) — Apply mineral oil to the silk just inside the tip of each ear. Use half to three-quarters of a medicine dropper's worth of the mineral oil in each ear. Do not apply the oil until the silk has wilted and begun to turn brown at the tip.

C

CORN (PLANTED) — Plant at least four rows of corn, no more than two and one-half feet apart to create better pollination.

Plant corn deeper than recommended to discourage crows.

CORNS — Make a poultice out of a quarter-cup of vinegar and crumbled bread. Let the mixture stand for forty-five minutes. Apply this poultice before going to bed. The next morning soreness should be gone, and the corn should be ready to be picked out. It may require more than one application.

After boiling a potato in its skin, take the skin and put the inside of it next to the corn. After the potato skin has been left on for twelve hours, the corn will be nearly cured.

If you are bothered by corns, drop a little vinegar on the corn and cover it with cooking soda. Let the mixture remain on the corn for ten minutes. Repeat six times a day, and in four days the corn will be gone. (This treatment will also work on warts.)

Rub corns with castor oil twice a day for four weeks.

White willow bark burned to ashes and steeped in vinegar takes away corns and other risings in the feet.

Place a piece of lemon peel on the corn. Put a Band-Aid around it to keep it in place.

Tape a moist teabag on the corn for forty-five minutes a day for seven days.

Wrap a piece of fresh pineapple peel (the inside of the peel next to the corn) around the corn. It should be gone within a week.

Bring five quarts of water to a boil. Add one and two-thirds cups of oatmeal. Boil until only four quarts of water remain. Strain and soak your feet in the water for twenty minutes.

COUGHING — To Cure: Place a small amount of dry pulverized borax on the tongue and let it slowly dissolve and run down the throat.

Combine one-half cup of apple-cider vinegar and one-half cup of water. Add one teaspoon of cayenne pepper and honey to taste. Take one tablespoon as needed and before bed.

Grate one teaspoon of horseradish. Add two teaspoons of honey. Take one teaspoon every two to three hours.

Squeeze the juice of one lemon into a glass. Add two tablespoons of honey, three whole cloves, and hot water. Drink one glass every three hours.

Cook a cup of barley according to the directions on the package. Add the juice of one lemon and some water. Liquefy in a blender. Drink one cup slowly every four hours.

Cut a hole almost through the middle of a yellow onion or a rutabaga. Fill with honey or brown sugar and leave overnight. In the morning, drink the juice.

Cut a hole in the middle of a large beet. Fill with honey or brown sugar. Bake until the beet is soft. Eat when you feel a cough coming on.

Add a one-inch piece of stick cinnamon, one tablespoon of honey, three to six cloves, and a few pieces of lemon peel to three cups of wine. Heat. Drink three cups every day.

For a dry cough, scrub three potatoes, then boil them with the skin on. Sweeten the water with honey. Take one tablespoon as needed.

Roast a lemon without burning it; when the lemon is thoroughly hot, cut it and squeeze the juice into a cup on three ounces of sugar, finely powdered. Take a teaspoon whenever cough troubles you.

Press hard on the roof of the mouth with your thumb.

Drink some anise tea.

Add a pinch of powdered quinine to a cup of water and drink.

Mix three drops of coal oil with a teaspoon of sugar. Take as needed.

Eat a mixture of vinegar and honey.

Heat the juice from two lemons. Do not boil, but be sure the juice is very hot. Pour it over three ounces of finely powdered sugar. Take one teaspoonful as needed.

For a cough or a tickling in the throat, take the juice of two lemons, the beaten white of one egg, and enough sugar to make a thick paste. A teaspoon of this mixture will ease the irritation and cure a cough in its early stages.

Cough Compound: For the cure of coughs, colds, asthma, whooping cough, and all diseases of the lungs, mix one spoonful of common tar, three spoons of honey, the yolks of three hen's eggs, and a half-pint of wine. Beat the tar, eggs, and honey well with a knife and bottle for use. Take a teaspoon every morning, noon, and night before eating.

Cough (Consumptive, To Cure): Take three pints of rain water, a half-pound of raisins chopped fine, and three tablespoons of flax seed. Sweeten to a syrup with honey and boil down to a quart. Add three teaspoons of extract of anise seed. Take a tablespoon eight times a day.

Cough Syrup: Boil the bark of a wild cherry tree in water. This syrup is also supposed to be good heart medicine.

Take two large Spanish onions and slice them thinly. Pour two cups of honey over them, cover, and let stand overnight. The next day strain off the syrup and add a jigger of brandy. Take one teaspoon of the syrup every three hours, keeping it bottled and refrigerated between uses.

Mix honey and horseradish together. Take as needed.

Mix one pint of whiskey with one-half pound of horehound candy.

Mix together the juice of one lemon, one cup of honey, and one-half cup of olive oil. Cook for five minutes. Take one teaspoon every two hours.

COW — During Pregnancy: Pour two ounces of apple-cider vinegar over the cow's feed two times a day. The calf will be on its feet five minutes after birth. It will nurse thirty minutes after birth.

To Test a Cow's Milk for Acid: Mix one tablespoon of soap powder with one quart of water (soap powder is very alkaline). Pour the mixture into a cup until it is one-third full. Next add four squirts of cow's milk from the teat. Swish the mixture around till it is thoroughly mixed. If the cow's milk is acid in reaction as it normally should be, the soap powder and water solution in the cup will be thinned and will pour like water from the cup. If the milk has changed to an alkaline reaction when it is poured, the solution will be thicker. It may be stringy as it is poured, or it may curdle in the cup.

To Relieve from Choking: If the object cannot be reached by two fingers of the hand inserted in the throat, the best means is to crush the obstacle by placing a block of wood on one side of the throat against it and striking a sharp blow on the other side with a wooden mallet. This will smash the object, and the cow can swallow it.

Kicking (To Cure): Put a garden hoe in front of the cow's hind leg and above and behind the gambrel joint of the nigh hind leg. Sit down on the right side to milk, and put the handle of the hoe well up under the arm and begin milking. The heifer cannot move either hind leg, and after one week she can be milked safely without fettering.

COW (TEA) — For a fertilizer and water mixture called "Cow Tea," put manure in a bucket of water and let it soak till the water is really dark. (Don't use any other chemicals.) Take a container such as a gallon milk jug, fill it with cow tea, twist a rag and push it to the bottom of the jug. Put the other end upside down, the jug into the ground near the bottom of the root system. (Keep the jug filled.)

COW (UDDER CAKED) — For swollen or caked udders on a cow, wash and rub the udders with water as hot as you can stand. Then rub with a dry cloth. Apply hog's lard, or, better, grate yellow carrot fine and simmer it in the lard to an ointment and apply and rub as above.

CRADLE CAP — Rub with vitamin-E oil.

CRAMP (WHILE BATHING OR SWIMMING) — Some people recommend a vigorous and violent shock to the part affected by suddenly and forcibly stretching out the leg, which should be darted out of the water into the air, if possible.

CRAYON (MARKS, REMOVING FROM PAINTED WALLS) — Put a little toothpaste on a dry rag, scrub off marks, and wipe with a damp cloth.

CRICKETS — Potatoes attract crickets.

CROPS (ESTIMATE) — Frame together four light sticks, measuring exactly a square foot inside. With this in one hand, walk into the field and select a spot of fair average yield; lower the frame square over as many heads as it will enclose. Shell out the heads enclosed carefully and weigh the grain. That proportion should be 43,560th part of an acre's production. To prove it, go through the field and make ten or twenty similar calculations and estimate by the mean of the whole number of results. This will enable a farmer to make closer calculations than he or she can by guessing.

CROPS (HARVEST) – Harvest all root crops in the late afternoon. Top crops should be harvested between ten in the morning and three in the afternoon.

CROUP (KRUP) – Drink the juice out of a roasted onion.

Mix honey and turpentine together and sip.

Wring a towel out well in ice water. Then place it around the throat and cover with a dry towel. Hold this in place until the towel begins to feel warm and then allow it to remain on for about twenty minutes. (Hundreds have written me to say how well this works.)

As soon as the first symptoms are discovered, apply cold water suddenly and freely to the neck and chest with a sponge, then lay a cloth wet with cold water on the chest and closely cover it with cotton batting (nothing else will do as well). Breathing will be instantly relieved. Give the patient plenty of cold water to drink and cover him or her warmly in bed. There is no danger of taking cold by this method.

Make a bib out of a piece of chamois skin. Melt together some tallow and pine tar and rub this in the chamois. Let the child with croup wear this all the time. The tar must be renewed occasionally.

Bind strips of flannel dipped in hot water about the throat. When the strips get cold, remove them and apply others that are hot.

CUCUMBER VINES – When you remove a cucumber from the vine, cut it with a knife, leaving about an eighth of an inch of the cucumber on the vine. Then slit the stem with a knife from its end to the vine, leaving a small portion of the cucumber on each division. Then on each division there will be a new cucumber as big as the first.

CURTAINS (TO MEND) – If one of your fine curtains develops a hole, you can do a neat job of "invisible mending" by covering the hole with a piece of white paper, then running the area back and forth under the sewing machine needle. After the curtain is laundered, the paper will have been soaked away and the darning will be hard to detect.

CUTS AND WOUNDS – Apply a slice of bread that has been soaked in milk. Wrap with a cloth.

Sprinkle black pepper on a thin slice of salt-pork fat and tie it very tightly against the wound.

Put a slice of tomato over the wound.

C

Apply sugar and bandage.

Apply a "fresh" spiderweb.

Apply vitamin-E oil.

Warm a small amount of spirits of turpentine. Pour it on the wound. Relief will come fast.

Cover a cut with flour to stop bleeding.

Apply aloe vera juice to a cut to stop the pain.

CUTWORMS – Keep the garden clear of weeds and grass through the fall months. This will discourage egg-laying cutworm moths. Sunflowers should be grown around the border of the garden. They repel cutworms. Place a stiff, three-inch-high collar of cardboard around stems of young plants. Push the collar down one inch into the soil.

Place crushed eggshells, damp wood ashes, or a mulch of oak leaves around each plant.

Scatter cornmeal around each plant. They may die of indigestion because cornmeal is a food that cutworms cannot digest.

Combine equal amounts of wheat bran and hardwood sawdust, and add enough molasses and water to make a sticky substance. Scatter this substance around each plant at dusk. This will cling to the bodies of the cutworms as they crawl around. It will soon harden, rendering them helpless.

CYSTS – Apply vitamin-E wheat-germ ointment.

Apply vitamin-E oil.

Eat a high-fiber diet.

Mix one tablespoon of castor oil with one-half teaspoon of baking soda and apply.

Make raw leafy vegetables the main part of your diet.

Eat seafood.

Avoid red meats, pork, and starches.

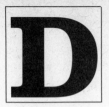

DAISIES — When you see a lot of daisies, the soil lacks lime.

DANDELIONS — Dandelions heat the soil by transporting minerals, especially calcium, upward from deep layers, even from underneath hardpan.

DANDRUFF — Dampen the scalp with sulphur water four times a week.

Use two thimblefuls of powdered refined borax. Let it dissolve in a teacup of water; next brush the head well, then wet a brush and apply it to the mixture and then to the head. Do this every day for ten days, then twice a week for three weeks.

Fill a quart bottle to a depth of one inch with borax. Fill the rest with water. Massage the scalp once a day with this mixture.

Mix three quarts of boiling water with two ounces of camomile and a two-and-one-half-inch ginger root, coarsely grated. Let this mixture stand until cool, then pour it into a smaller container. Massage the head with this mixture twice a day for three days.

The desert's amole or yucca root, when made into a sudsy shampoo, will eliminate dandruff.

Pour some warm cider vinegar on your hair, then wrap a towel around your head. Leave the towel on for one hour. After the hour is up, wash your head. Do this three times a week for a month. Your dandruff will disappear.

Don't use refined sugar. Sweeten with honey.

Take brewer's yeast.

Wash your hair in one cup of beet juice mixed with two cups of water and one teaspoon of salt. (Note: This could darken the hair of light-haired people.)

Squeeze the juice of one lemon and apply half of it to your hair. Then wash your hair with a mild shampoo and rinse with water. Mix the other half of the lemon juice with two cups of water and rinse your hair with this. Repeat every other day until the dandruff is gone.

Massage the head with a mixture of one pint of boiling water mixed with two tablespoons of dried rosemary soaked for three hours.

DDT — DDT and other pesticides go straight to the seed oil of corn or cotton. There is no way to remove them. Use cold-processed oils, such as olive oil or safflower oil.

DECONGESTANT — Smoke mullein.

D

DEFROSTER — Here's a cheap "defroster" that keeps snow, sleet, and ice from forming on your windshield. Rub a little moistened salt on the outside of the windshield and renew the treatment as necessary. Before driving off in winter, store a box of fine-grain salt in your glove compartment.

DENTAL PROBLEMS — Massaging the area of your hand between the thumb and index finger can help relieve a toothache.

To prevent tooth decay in children, never allow your child to sleep with a bottle containing milk, formula, fruit juice, or other sweet liquids.

To speed healing after dental surgery, eat pineapple every day for a few days before your operation. After your operation, drink pineapple juice until you are again able to eat the fruit itself.

Take zinc supplements immediately before and after dental surgery.

Rub peppermint oil on your gums to relieve pain.

Rinse your mouth with Epsom salt and hot water.

DEODORIZER — Burn some sugar on hot coals.

Roast coffee, finely ground, on an iron plate.

For a bathroom deodorizer, strike a match, then drop it in the toilet stool.

For a sickroom deodorizer, sprinkle vinegar all along the baseboard.

DEPRESSION — Eat two ripe bananas a day.

Make love.

Eat a lot of mint.

Confine yourself to an air-conditioned house for four days and take regular ten-minute cold showers.

Be sure every room is well lighted.

Take long walks.

Eat properly and get plenty of rest.

Eat watercress, spinach, and carrots.

Pets can help people overcome depression.

Exercising each day also helps combat depression.

DIABETES — Eat sunchokes (Jerusalem artichokes).

Yucca root, mashed and boiled, makes an effective tea.

Eat one-quarter of a medium-sized raw potato daily.

Eat one piece of celery daily.

DIAMOND (TO TEST AUTHENTICITY) — Immerse the diamond or artificial stone in alcohol or water. The diamond will not lose its lustre. The artificial stone will. Touch the diamond to your tongue. It will feel cold; glass, much less so.

DIAPER (PINS) — Diaper pins can be sharpened just by running them through a hair-filled pin cushion a few times. It will also keep them from rusting.

DIAPER RASH — Apply liquid lecithin.

Apply vitamin-E oil.

DIARRHEA — **Acute:** Eat strained carrots or carrot soup.

Drink rice water daily (adults — one-half cup twice a day; babies — two teaspoons in a bottle of milk twice a day).

Eat bananas, carrots, and lots of yogurt.

Grate some raw apples and wait until they turn dark. Eat as many of the grated apples as you feel like.

Beat the white of an egg until it is frothy. Add the juice of half a lemon. Drink.

Drink two tablespoons of blackberry brandy every four hours.

Eat cooked rice with a dash of cinnamon.

Add one teaspoon of chopped garlic to one teaspoon of honey. Take three times a day, two hours after each meal.

Mix one tablespoon of flour with eight ounces of water and drink.

Bacterial: Drink eight ounces of blackberry juice or four ounces of blackberry wine every four hours.

Four times a day eat one ripe banana that has been soaked in milk.

Drink buttermilk.

Eat raw sauerkraut, yogurt, or pickled beets.

DIETS — **How to diet:** First day — Eat all the raw apples you want.

Second day — Eat three balanced meals.

Third day — All the apples you want.

Fourth day — Three balanced meals.

At the end of each day, take two tablespoons of olive oil. Keep this up for twenty days, and you should be able to see the results. If satisfied with this diet at the end of twenty days, keep doing it in the same manner. After reaching your desired weight, start eating regular meals each day, but keep from eating too much.

Remember, watch out for fad diets. Also, don't be a girdle prisoner. The food choices we make today will tell us what we will be in fifteen to twenty years. Remember that we are preparing our own fates.

A British experiment proves that 90 percent of each pound lost is fat, not water, after the initial week of dieting.

DIETS (FRYMIRE'S POTATO) — Do the following daily: Cut one medium-sized raw potato into four equal pieces. Eat one piece twenty to thirty minutes before breakfast; one, twenty to thirty minutes before lunch; another, twenty to thirty minutes before supper. Never eat supper later than 6:00 P.M. Eat the last piece of the potato at 8:00 P.M. Eat three regular meals daily and, please, no snacks. Place the unused potato pieces in water and store in the refrigerator.

DIPLODIA (TWIG BLIGHT) — When the tips of your Scotch pine trees turn brown, it is probably caused by a condition called Diplodia twig blight. Affected tissues should be pruned and destroyed.

DIGESTIVE PROBLEMS AND NAUSEA — Drink cinnamon water and slacked lime (lime-water).

DISEASES (CHILDHOOD, TREATMENT OF) — A baby not yet able to talk must cry when it is ill. Colic makes a baby cry loudly and shed tears, stopping for a moment and beginning again. If the chest is affected, it gives one sharp cry, breaking off immediately, as if crying hurt it. If the head is affected, it cries in sharp, piercing shrieks, with low moans and wails between. Or there may be periods of quiet dozing with wakefulness between.

It is easy to perceive when a child is attacked by disease that there is some change taking place. Either the skin will be dry and hot or the appetite gone. The baby will be sleepy or fretful and crying. It will be thirsty and pale. When a child vomits or has diarrhea or is feverish, it is due to some illness and needs attention. These various symptoms may continue for a day or two before the disease can be diagnosed. A warm bath, warm drinks, etc., can do no harm and may help to determine the cause of the discomfort.

On coming out of the bath and being well rubbed with the hand, the baby will develop a rash if the problem is a skin disease. The appearance of the rash will help determine the specific disease. If the disease is scarlet fever, the skin will look deep pink all over the body, but mostly about the neck and face. Chicken pox shows fever, but not much of a runny nose or cold symptoms, as in measles, nor is there much of a cough. The spots are smaller and do not run much together, but are more spread out over the body and enlarge into blisters in a day or two.

Keep sick children in a shady, quiet, and cool room. Do not speak suddenly to startle a half-sleeping patient and handle the child with care when it is necessary to move him or her. If the lungs suffer, elevate the child on pillows for easier breathing, and do everything to soothe and make the child comfortable so he or she won't cry and distress inflamed lungs. If the child is very weak, do not move him or her suddenly to avoid startling the patient into convulsions. In bathing, greatest pains should be taken not to frighten the child. Place him or her gradually into the water and be amused by something to reassure the child that water is nothing to be afraid of. Keep up a good supply of fresh air at about sixty-six degrees Fahrenheit. If you must have a hired nurse, select one who is intelligent, gentle, loving, and kind, with good manners and a pleasant temperament. Your child will be safe in the presence of such a person. The nurse should not be under twenty-five or over fifty-five so as to be at her full strength and capacity.

DISINFECTANTS — Cut good-sized onions in halves, and place them on a plate on the floor. They will absorb odors in a short time. Change to newly sliced onions every five hours.

DIZZINESS — Try taking deep breaths and, as you exhale, count slowly in a voice that you can understand. Do this several times each day. You will be pleased with the results.

A simple change in diet sometimes helps alleviate dizziness.

DOG — A dog who lives outdoors all year needs more food in winter than in hot months. Also include extra fat in its diet.

DOG DAYS — Dog days in the South will begin on July 28 and continue on to September 5. In the North and East, dog days begin on July 3 and continue until August 11. It is the one season of the year that calls for a measure of toleration rather than celebration.

Grain bins and barn lofts are more likely to cave in during this period.

DOG PROBLEMS — **Skin Problems:** If a dog has eczema, mix two tablespoons of cottage cheese and two tablespoons of corn oil. Add to this mixture five or six drops of vitamin E and one capsule of garlic. Add this to the dog's food daily.

Rub the dog's coat with liquid vitamin E twice a day.

For every ten pounds of the dog's weight, put one tablespoon of safflower oil in its food and mix well.

Give the dog soybean, peanut, and safflower oils.

Once a day, for every sixty pounds of the dog's weight, give it a four-hundred-I.U. capsule of vitamin E, a heaping tablespoon of brewer's yeast, and one-half teaspoon of cod-liver oil.

Give the dog ten milligrams of zinc each day.

Fleas and Ticks: Give brewer's yeast to the dog (at the rate of one rounded tablespoon per fifty pounds of body weight) and fresh garlic.

Add cooked grains, such as rolled oats, cornmeal, and bran to the dog's food once a day.

For every ten pounds of weight, give one garlic capsule every other day.

If cedar shavings are used in a dog's bed, there will be no fleas since fleas will not tolerate the aroma of cedar.

D

Canine Seizures: Crush some sunflower seeds and put them in the dog's food.

Give one vitamin-E pill daily.

Give a puppy a B-complex vitamin and dolomite powder twice a day.

Lameness and Arthritis: Give a bone-meal tablet, one tablet for a large dog and a quarter tablet for a very small dog.

Give vitamin E for ten days.

Give twenty alfalfa tablets each day for ninety days.

Sores: Give the dog desiccated-liver tablets for ten days.

For a collie, give four of the ten-grain tablets of brewer's yeast for two weeks.

Worms: Give puppies a clove of garlic, raw and chopped fine, in the food once a week. Give two capsules of garlic for seven days and then one every other day for older dogs.

Wetting on Furniture and Carpets: Place or shake black pepper around your furniture legs and on carpets. Vacuum up the pepper after four to seven days.

Place some paper where you would like your dog to go. At the edge of the paper place a very small bed of cedar shavings.

DOUGHNUTS — Sugar doughnuts easily and quickly by placing them in a paper bag with a small quantity of powdered sugar. Then shake.

DOWSING — Witching or dowsing for underground water, oil, minerals, and other things is a gift. If you have it, you will be willing to concentrate and do the following:

1) Place a piece of string or rope on the floor in front of you.

2) Place a wire coat hanger in each hand with the hanger part pointing up.

3) Concentrate on the rope in front of you and slowly walk toward it. The coat hangers should swing in or out when you get to the rope. Usually, it won't take longer than two hours of practice to be able to do this.

4) After mastering this part, you are now ready for the supreme test.

5) Have someone blindfold you and place the piece of rope in a different place in front of you.

6) Have someone place the coat hangers in your hands with the hanger part pointing up and then point you in the direction of the rope.

7) When you get to the piece of rope that was stretched out in front of you, the coat hangers will swing in or out. Surprise, you did it!

All this takes a little practice, patience, and lots of concentration. But you are ready to dowse for anything once you have mastered this procedure.

DRAIN (PREVENT CLOGGING) — Pour one cup of baking soda into the drain every week. Follow it with one cup of vinegar. As the soda and vinegar foam up, flush the drain with a quart of boiling water.

DRAIN CLEANER — Mix a cup each of salt and baking soda with one-quarter cup of cream of tartar. Be sure to mix well. Put one-quarter cup of the mix in a drain, following it with a cup of boiling water. Wait thirty seconds and flush with cold water.

Keep sinks, drains, and tubs free of grease and disagreeable odors by pouring ordinary hot saltwater through them once or twice a week.

DRINKER (SOCIAL) — If the social drinker who occasionally has one too many thinks the room is spinning, have him or her lie on a bed and put a foot on the floor.

Have a person who has had too much to drink eat cucumbers.

Massage the tip of the drunk person's nose.

Give the drunk person a teaspoon of honey every few minutes.

Have the drunk eat a handful of raw almonds.

Have him or her eat cabbage with a little vinegar on it.

Administer one teaspoon of the following mixture two times a day: sulphate of iron, twenty grains; peppermint, forty-four drams; magnesia, forty grains; spirits of nutmeg, four drams.

To diminish the effects of alcohol, eat one cup of raw sauerkraut. Drinking a glass of milk with nutmeg in it also may help.

DROPSY — Dig some silkweed or milkweed roots, make tea out of them, and drink it.

Make a tea out of chestnut leaves. Drink this in place of water, and it should cure you in a few days.

DYSENTERY — Take one egg and beat slightly; if desired, add a pinch of sugar. Swallow the egg at a gulp. Do this two or three times a day. Stay quiet. Recovery should be rather rapid.

For bacterial dysentery, eat a finely chopped raw onion in a cup of yogurt daily.

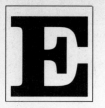

EAR (NOISES) — To help alleviate noises in the ear, avoid alcohol, nicotine, marijuana, caffeine, aspirin products, prescription tranquilizers, oral contraceptives, quinine, overdoses of vitamin D, and overexposure to the sun. You should also avoid exposure to extremely loud noises.

Daily zinc supplements can also help ear noises.

The problem may be caused by manganese deficiency. Manganese is found in whole-grain products, fruits (especially bananas), eggs, vegetables (especially legumes), liver, and other organ meats.

A deficiency of choline may also be the cause of the problem. Choline is found in lecithin, soybeans, eggs, fish, liver, wheat germ, green vegetables, peanuts, brewer's yeast, and sunflower seeds.

To mask the noise within your ears, try keeping a radio on.

EAR (PROBLEMS) — To prevent itchy ears, apply baby oil, petroleum jelly, or glycerine to your ear with your little finger. Never use cotton-tipped applicators.

Make sure that soap and shampoo do not get into your ears. If they do, be sure to rinse your ears.

Do not swim in ponds or slow-moving bodies of water.

Completely dry your ears after swimming.

Try this solution after swimming: mix two tablespoons of boiled water with thirty drops of white vinegar. Let the mixture cool before using it. Apply two or three drops in each ear.

EAR (RINGING) — This problem could be caused by overusing aspirin or other drugs.

Place two drops of onion juice in each ear four times a week.

Place a heating pad on your feet and hands.

Place a paper bag over your head; breathe in and out twenty times. Do this three times daily.

Mix one tablespoon of cider vinegar and one tablespoon of honey with eight ounces of water. Take three times daily.

Gently rub the tips of your fingers together for two minutes. Do this three times daily. In ten days you should see improvement.

In a circular motion, massage over each eye on the forehead for two minutes. Do this twice daily.

Eat one banana a day.

If the ringing persists, seek medical attention.

EAR (TROUBLE: INFECTION AND WAX BUILD-UP) — Mix equal parts of white vinegar and rubbing alcohol. Flush ears as needed.

To combat wax build-up in ears, put eight drops of warm hydrogen peroxide in the ear and let it fizz for two minutes. Then tilt your head so that the liquid runs out onto a tissue. Remove the wax with soft cotton.

EARACHE — Into an iron pan, place some live coals, sprinkle the coals with brown sugar, and invert a funnel over the live coals and brown sugar. Place the end of the funnel in your ear. The smoke will give relief.

Mix one grain of chloroform and one ounce of olive oil and shake well together. Then pour twenty drops in the affected ear and insert a piece of cotton. The relief should be prompt. If further treatment is needed, rub the back of the ear with warm laudanum. In case of discharge from the ear, carefully syringe the ear with warm water and milk.

Combine five drops of onion juice with one teaspoon of warm olive oil. Put three drops in each ear twice a day. Plug the ears with cotton.

Sprinkle castor-oil cotton with black pepper and apply to the aching ear.

ECZEMA — Eat two raw potatoes a day for ten days.

Take thirty milligrams of zinc a day.

Take six zinc tablets a day along with vitamin A.

Some people take zinc, fifty milligram doses, three times a day.

Take two brewer's yeast tablets three times a day.

Do not eat fried foods, white bread, potatoes, or beef.

Do not drink beer or carbonated beverages.

Massage the spine with a mixture of one teaspoon of castor oil and two pinches of sulphur.

Eat a high-fiber diet and lots of vegetables.

Try taking two teaspoons of blackstrap molasses in a glass of milk twice a day.

Boiled jimson weed with cooked slippery elm bark spread on a cloth and tied around the affected area seems to help. Never take jimson weed internally because it is poisonous.

E

Try two tablespoons of safflower oil daily to get rid of eczema.

EGGS — Boiled carrots are an excellent substitute for eggs in pudding. Be sure to mash the boiled carrots and press them through a coarse cloth or strainer. This will produce pulp.

Old eggs are smooth and shiny. Fresh eggs are rough and chalky in appearance.

Quickly and easily separate the whites from the yolks of eggs by breaking them gently into a funnel. The whites pass through and the yolks remain. (Note: It's easiest to separate whites and yolks right after removing the eggs from the refrigerator.)

Don't wash eggs before storing. Water destroys the protective film that keeps out air and odors.

Generations of doctors have found eggs valuable in preventing and treating both tuberculosis and rheumatic fever. Eggs are very digestible. Nothing is more healing and comforting than a couple of poached or soft-boiled eggs on milk toast.

Eggs are good for your nerves and brain. Have you ever wondered why, if they weren't good for you, God would have put so important a substance in so precious a container? Eggs provide energy without a lot of calories.

Add a few drops of vinegar to water in which eggs are being boiled. It will keep the shells from cracking and the whites from oozing out.

To test the age of an egg, put it in a deep container of cold water. A fresh egg will lie on its side at the bottom of the water. An egg that inclines at an angle is several days old. An egg that stands upright is about a week and a half old. An egg that floats to the top is too old to use.

Egg whites can be used to mend a tear. Spread egg white on the wrong side of the fabric when it is laid flat. Cover the rip with a linen scrap larger than the tear and press with a hot iron.

To keep egg yolks fresh for several days, cover them with cold water and store in the refrigerator.

Easter eggs won't crack if you place a needle hole in one end so that air can escape.

EMOTIONAL PROBLEMS — Lay off the sweets.

Drink distilled water only.

Sometimes eating hot dogs will trigger emotional problems related to allergies.

ETIQUETTE (TABLE) — The first thing to do is to sit down and think how you really behave at the table. Are your hands, nails, and face clean? Is your hair brushed back smoothly? Do you seat yourself quietly and remember to put your napkin on your lap? Do you sometimes put your knife in your mouth instead of your fork or spoon? Do you pour your tea in your saucer instead of drinking it from the cup? How do you pass your plate if you are to be helped a second time? The best way is to hold your knife and fork in your hand. That way they won't fall onto the tablecloth.

Then think about passing food. Do you reach over another person's plate or stand up to reach something not near and knock over a glass or cruet in your attempt? Do you eat fast and loud, put large pieces in your mouth, speak with food unchewed, or pick your teeth? Remember not to whisper, yawn, or stretch, touch your hair, or blow your nose. If it is necessary to use your handkerchief, do so quietly so that no one will notice. Ideally, you should use your handkerchief before coming to the table. If there are bones, cherry pits, and things that cannot be swallowed, put them on your spoon, then on your plate.

EXERCISE (FOR YOUR BACK) — Lie flat on your back. Tuck your toes under the side of a bed or sofa. Clasp your hands behind your neck. Now do twelve or fifteen sit-ups. Do this twice a day.

To ease lower back pain, lie flat on your back. Keeping your legs straight, raise your hips and knees to a forty-five-degree angle and sit up. This will be hard to do. Do it twenty-five times daily.

Don't forget that neck tension can affect your back. Do my neck exercises: Stretch your neck to full capacity, roll it in a wide circle four times clockwise, then four times counterclockwise. Tilt your head to the left four times, then to the right four times. Next tilt your head backward four times, forward four times. Do this twice daily.

Always exercise for a few minutes daily.

Do not sit in the same chair twice in a row. Change from one chair to another.

While working, take three-minute breaks for walking and stretching.

If you drive long distances, stop often and relax.

What might be adequate exercise for one individual might be inadequate for another.

EYES — For black or sore eyes, make a poultice of a scraped raw potato.

If you have a cinder in your eye, chop up an onion and let your tears wash the cinder away.

For eye irritations, place a raw potato poultice on the eye. Leave it on for twenty minutes twice daily.

To treat pink eye, place an apple poultice on the eye for forty-five minutes.

If your eyes are puffy, apply used tea bags (moist and cool) to the closed eyelids for fifteen minutes.

Another treatment is to take one-half ounce of watermelon seed daily. Make this by pouring boiling water over a level teaspoon of crushed seed and steeping for thirty minutes.

Eating carrots, celery, lettuce, and mustard greens with lemon juice may also help.

You should avoid meat, wine, and carbonated drinks.

Place slices of cucumber or potato on closed eyes to reduce puffiness and bags under the eyes.

To treat a sty, moisten a non-herbal tea bag, put it over the closed eye, bandage it in place, and leave on overnight.

For sunburned eyes, apply a poultice of grated apples to the eyes and leave it for an hour. Or apply a poultice of lightly beaten egg white to your eyes and leave overnight.

Willow-bark extract is helpful in cleansing and healing inflamed and infected eyes.

To remove small objects from the eyes, take a horsehair and double it. This will leave a loop. If the object can be seen, lay the loop over it, then close the eye. The object will come out as the hair is withdrawn.

To strengthen your eyesight, place a little pressure on the eyeballs with your finger. The pressure must be from the nose to the temples. Wash the eyes three times daily with cold water.

You can prevent your eyes from watering while you are peeling onions by placing a small piece of polished steel or a needle between the teeth while you peel. The polished steel or needle will attract the acid juice of the onion.

As a remedy for weak eyes, mix a weak brandy and water lotion. Keep this solution ready-mixed in a bottle. Mix just enough brandy with the water to cause a slight sensation when you apply the mixture to the eyes.

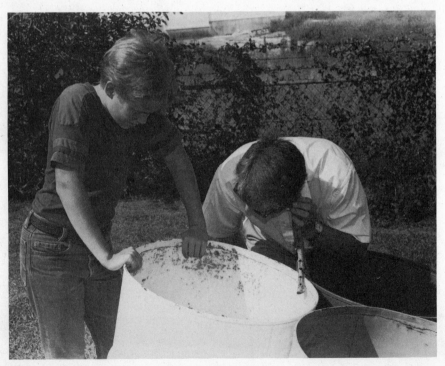

**Frymire's
Earthquake Device**

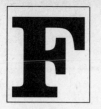

FACE (CLEAN) — Mix one-half cup of cornmeal and one-half cup of oatmeal with just enough milk or cream to make a paste. Apply the paste to your face and massage well. Wash off with warm water after thirty minutes.

FACE (SHAVE) — Shave sometime during the morning hours for one week, during the afternoon the next week. Alternate back and forth. On Tuesday of each week, shave mornings and at night. Rub on some Listerine after shaving. If you plan to shave just once a week, Tuesday is the best day.

FAINTING — Give the person who faints due to heart trouble a tumbler of equal parts cold brandy and water.

Try having a person who has regular fainting spells sniff black pepper.

FAITHFULNESS — To make sure that your future husband or wife will be faithful, you must both lick your thumbs. Then press them together in a promise of faithfulness.

FATIGUE — Drink ginseng tea.

Mix two tablespoons of apple-cider vinegar and one teaspoon of honey with one cup of warm water. Drink a cup of this tonic every morning before breakfast. Be sure to sip it slowly.

Drink a cup of water to which one-eighth of a teaspoon of cayenne pepper has been added.

Every morning and evening walk barefoot in dewy grass for five to ten minutes.

To combat mental fatigue, cut an unpeeled apple into small pieces and place them in a bowl. Add two cups of boiling water and let the mixture steep for one hour. Then add one tablespoon of honey. Drink the water and eat the pieces of apple.

FAUCETS — To remove brown spots from around faucets, clean them with a mixture of vinegar (or lemon juice) and water. Rinse with clean water.

FEET — **Aching:** Sprinkle cayenne pepper on your socks or rub it directly onto your feet.

Soak your feet in hot water for fifteen minutes. Then massage them with lemon juice. Rinse with cool water, and take five deep breaths.

Do this simple massage for aching feet standing or sitting. Take a shoebox and fill it with one layer of marbles. Rub one foot at a time over the marbles at whatever pressure feels best for as long as you like. Be sure the marbles have plenty of room for movement.

To restore life to sore feet, mix one cup of salt in one gallon of very warm water. Soak your feet in this mixture till the water cools. Rub your feet while they are in the water. Dry them thoroughly and rub them well with a good towel. Be sure the water-and-salt mixture covers the ankles. You may have to use two cups salt and two gallons of water.

To relieve foot fatigue while walking, pick some ferns and stuff these into your shoes or boots. This should provide refreshing and quick relief for sore and tired feet.

For pain in the heel, walk more and do stretching exercises. Place a heel pad in your shoe.

Burning: Wrap tomato slices on the bottom of each foot and keep them elevated for forty-five minutes. Do this three times a day.

Boil five scrubbed potatoes in a pan with three quarts of water until the potatoes are soft. Remove the potatoes. Let the water cool a little, then soak your feet in it for twenty minutes. Dry the feet thoroughly and, if you are going to bed, massage them with almond oil. Sleep in loose-fitting socks to avoid messing up the sheets.

Some people, after they have soaked their feet in potato water, sprinkle hot, roasted salt on a cloth and wrap it around their feet.

Perspiring, Smelly Feet: To keep feet from perspiring, bathe them each night in a strong solution of borax. It may take three weeks to cure the problem.

Dust the inside of your shoes with borax.

Put ten drops of distilled turpentine in a container of two gallons of hot water. Submerge the feet in the water until it becomes cool or room temperature, then remove the feet but do not dry them off with a towel. Allow them to dry on their own. Repeat this solution for seven days, then every other day for a week, then once the following week.

Scaly, Itchy Feet: This problem is often caused by eczema of the feet and is usually noticed right after you start wearing a new pair of shoes that have rubber soles. This rubber has been sanitized with a chemical called mercaptobezthiazole. Many people are allergic to this chemical. If you are bothered by this problem, get rid of the shoes and buy leather-soled ones. You will also have to get rid of the socks that you wore in the rubber-soled shoes.

Protect your feet from moisture by giving the soles of your shoes several coats of shellac.

FEMALE PROBLEMS (FRIGIDITY) — To overcome a lack of lust, a woman should mix one teaspoon of powdered licorice with a cup of water and drink it. Do this daily.

Another treatment is to mix sesame seeds with honey and take two tablespoons daily.

You can also try gently massaging the back of the leg near the ankle. This will relax tension, stimulate circulation, and soothe the female organs.

Take cabbage-rose leaves (or any common red-rose leaves will do) and put them in a china teapot. Use one-half ounce of leaves and cover them with one pint of boiling water. Let the mixture stand for ten minutes, then pour off the water. Let it get cold and then sweeten it with sugar or honey. A wine glass full of this drink taken occasionally will usually help.

FENCE POST (TO KEEP FROM ROTTING) — Take boiled linseed oil and stir it into pulverized charcoal to create the consistency of paint. Put a coat of this on the posts.

FERTILITY (REMEDY) — Drink wild ginseng tea.

Robitussin cough syrup will help some women overcome fertility problems.

FEVER — Plain aspirin can be taken to reduce fever but do not use an aspirin compound that contains caffeine.

Children should be given acetaminophen. Do not give a feverish child aspirin.

Drink at least two quarts of water or juice a day. Do not drink anything that contains caffeine, which can increase body temperature.

For an especially high fever, try the following:
    Bind peeled garlic cloves or sliced onions to the bottoms of the feet.
    Sip diluted pure grape juice throughout the day. Drink it at room temperature, not chilled.
    Eat grapes throughout the day.
    Sip some hot spicebush tea.

Lie down on a pile of cool willow leaves. When the leaves become warm, it is believed that the fever has been transferred to them.

Drink three cups of dittany tea. (Some people call the dittany plant a fever plant.)

Drink Wahoo tea.

Drink a cupful of hard cider.

FEVER BLISTERS — Get oil from behind the ear and rub on the blister.

Drink buttermilk.

Eat three almonds daily.

Eat one-half cup raw sauerkraut daily.

Eat a high-fiber diet.

Apply Listerine.

Apply lemon juice.

Do not eat acidic foods or high-fat foods to prevent or reduce the length of duration of fever blisters. Eat plenty of alkaline foods and take B-complex vitamins. You should also avoid stress, sunburn, emotional upsets, colds, and fever.

Vitamin E applied to fever blisters should help to heal them faster and reduce the pain.

An ice cube applied to a fever blister for forty-five minutes should help.

F

Apply camphor or phenol lotion to fever blisters to shrink them and reduce the pain.

FEVER (DRINK) — Weak green tea with lemon juice added, taken hot, makes a good fever drink.

FEVER (HAY) — This problem can be relieved by bathing the nose and closed eyes with a lotion of spirits of camphor and warm water. The proper strength of the lotion will soon be determined from experience. The eyes must be carefully closed.

Eat two teaspoons of local raw honey twice a day.

Chew some honeycomb for twenty minutes at the start of a hay-fever attack. This should bring relief. After chewing the waxy stuff, throw it out.

Eat strawberries, grapes, and prunes.

Take a teaspoonful of grated orange or lemon peel sweetened with a little honey.

Pick a pint of tender ragweed leaves. Place them in a pan with a pint of distilled water. Let them simmer until half of the water has cooked off. Strain the remainder and add one-half cup of grain alcohol. Stir well and give the hay-fever sufferer one teaspoon a day during July, August, and September.

FIGS — Mix figs, dates, and cornmeal or crushed wheat and cook. Eat daily.

FINGERNAILS — Clay poultices can help split nails grow out healthy.

Vitamin-E oil also helps nails grow correctly.

Zinc can help clear up fungal infections under nails. Try three tablets a day.

For splitting nails, soak hands or nails in saltwater twice a day for twenty minutes each time.

Massage nails with castor oil once a day and leave the oil on for five to ten minutes. Then wipe nails off.

Soak your fingernails in warm Epsom-salt water to help splitting, layering, and chipping.

If you are bothered by brittle nails, tap them on a hard surface every chance you get. This will toughen them up.

Take iron supplements for brittle nails.

Apply liquid Micatin three times daily for fungus.

The Fry-Son Sleeper made from four paper clips and five rubber bands seems to help fingernails when it is used according to instructions. (See page 165 for instructions.)

Cut your nails nine Sundays in a row, and you will find a mate.

FISH — To improve the quality of your frozen fish, squeeze lemon juice over them before packaging them for the freezer.

To preserve fish for transporting, stop up the mouth of the fish with breadcrumbs soaked in a very small amount of brandy. Use clean straw to pack the fish.

Leaving fresh fish in water makes for poorer flavor.

Completely thawing frozen fish before cooking removes the flavor and nutriments.

Skinning a frozen fish after it is gutted is easier than doing it when it is fresh.

Fresh-caught fish should be cooked or frozen the day you catch them or the next day at the latest.

To check the freshness of fish in the store, be sure that the flesh is firm and springs back when touched. Eyes should be bright and clear. Scales should be anchored to the skin, and the fish should have either no odor or a pleasant, briny scent. A fish with a strong odor is too old to buy; when cooked, it will taste the way it smells.

FISHING (TRIP) — When planning a fishing trip, watch and see if the cattle are grazing. If they are, the fish will be biting too.

FITS (TREATMENT FOR THOSE CAUSED BY INDIGESTION) — Place the affected child in a warm bath at once. Give the child warm water and rub him or her briskly.

FLEAS (IN HOUSE) — Place pieces of walnut tree limbs throughout the house.

Close the house and put mothball flakes generously on the floor in every room. The house has to be closed for at least four days. The mothball flakes put the fleas to sleep for good, and the flakes will dissolve.

FLIES (TO DESTROY) — Mix half a teaspoon of black pepper, one teaspoon of brown sugar, and one tablespoon of cream. Be sure to mix well. Place this mixture in a room on a plate where flies are troublesome. Bye-bye, flies.

FLOUR — You won't waste flour if you dust it from a large salt shaker onto meats, fish, or patties instead of dipping the food into the flour. It's easier, too.

FLOWERS (CUT) — Cut flowers will keep longer if the leaves below the water are removed. Decaying vegetable matter poisons the water.

Don't discard fading flowers, but don't let them stand around half dead. Dispose of the withered blooms, rearranging the others with some greens in a smaller container to make them look as attractive as possible.

Cut flowers arrange very nicely if the bowl they are in is filled with hair rollers wired together with plastic ties.

Keep cut flowers fresh by adding a lump of sugar or camphor to the water.

Plunge cut flowers in warm water, not cold. Moisture is best absorbed by the stems at about one hundred degrees Fahrenheit. Flowers like cool heads but warm feet.

FLU — Anyone too ill to keep water down should drink peach juice. (This also works for teething babies.)

Apply an onion poultice over the throat and chest. An onion poultice placed over the neck, the back of the head, and the pit of the stomach also works. Leave these on for three hours.

FORECASTING — I think nature does know what she has in store. But I don't think mankind understands nature sufficiently to read the signs correctly.

If many snakes are plowed up in the fall, it means a mild winter. If none are plowed up, it means a bad winter.

If fish break water, a rainstorm is on the way.

By Small Animals: Winter will be bad if:
  1) squirrels build nests low in trees;
  2) the fur on animals such as dogs, sheep, horses, mules, and cows is thicker than usual;
  3) squirrels begin gathering nuts early (middle or late September);
  4) the fur on the bottoms of rabbits' feet is thicker;
  5) squirrels, rabbits, and possums have a thicker coat of fur than usual.
Animals act quite strangely before an earthquake.

By Birds: Birds fly higher in good weather.
  Birds fly close to the ground before a storm. Many will gather and roost, no matter what the time of day.
  If migrating geese fly due north or south, the next day will be fair. If they "tack" from east to west, the next day will bring bad weather.
  If the cuckoos do not cease singing at midsummer, corn will be dear.
  When the thrush sings at sunset, a fair day will follow.
  Magpies flying three or four together and uttering brash cries predict windy weather.
  Winter will be bad if:
  1) birds huddle on the ground;
  2) crows gather together;
  3) birds eat up all the berries early;
  4) hoot owls call late in fall;
  5) screech owls sound like women crying.
  If the breastbone of a turkey cooked in fall is white, it indicates that a mild winter is in store. If the turkey bone is purple or dark blue, a harsh winter is in store.
  Listen to the sparrows in the trees for an oncoming storm. They gather, and, if they have evergreen trees, they pack in and ride with the wind. Their chatter could drive a wooden man crazy if he had to stay outdoors within hearing distance of their din. They are very good short-range forecasters. If you hear them, prepare for a storm. It will arrive.

It's a sure sign of rain if hens gather on high ground and trim their feathers.

By Blasting Days: If it rains on "blasting days" (the three longest days of the year), there won't be any "mast" (acorns, chestnuts, etc.) for animals like hogs to feed on.

The weather will be fair if on blasting days:

> Smoke rises.
> You hear a screech owl.
> Crickets holler. (For this, the temperature will also rise.)

By Candlemas: When the blackbird sings before Christmas, she will cry before Candlemas (February 2).

A windy Christmas and a calm Candlemas are signs of a good year.

By Cattle: When cattle (or horses) lie with their heads upon the ground, it is a sign of rain.

If the bull leads the herd in going to pasture, rain must be expected. But if he is careless and allows cows to precede him, look for uncertain weather.

When a cow tries to scratch its ear, it means a shower is very near. When it thumps its ribs with its tail, look out for thunder, lightning, and hail.

Cows and deer stand facing west if bad weather is approaching. Good weather on the way or continuing means they will face east when they are standing.

By Christmas: Warm Christmas, cold Easter; green Christmas, white Easter.

A green Christmas makes a fat graveyard.

If ice will bear a man before Christmas, it will not bear a man afterward.

If the sun shines through the apple trees on Christmas day, there will be an abundant crop the following year.

Much ice on Christmas and New Year's Day is a sign of a big fruit crop.

A clear, bright sun on Christmas day foretells a peaceful year and plenty; but if the wind grows stormy before sunset, it betokens sickness in the spring and autumn quarters.

Light Christmas, light wheat sheaf (full moon near Christmas day); dark Christmas, heavy wheat sheaf.

A wet Christmas means an empty granary and barrel.

If it snows during Christmas night, the crops will do well.

So far as the sun shines on Christmas day, so far will the snow blow in May.

Snow on Christmas night means a good hop crop the next year.

If at Christmas ice hangs on the willow, clover may be cut at Easter.

If on Christmas night the wine ferments heavily in the barrels, a good wine year is to follow.

Thunder during Christmas week foretells much snow during the winter.

If it rains much during the twelve days after Christmas, expect a wet year.

A green Christmas means a hard and cold early spring.

The first twelve days after Christmas indicate what each month in the next year will be like.

F

By Fire: It will be a hard winter if smoke from the chimney flows toward or settles on the ground. It will snow within twenty-six days.

If noises that sound like boots swishing through dry, deep snow are coming from the chimney, there will be a deep snow.

If it's cloudy and smoke rises, there's a chance of snow.

When you build a fire outside and it pops, it will snow in three days.

Fire is said to burn brighter and throw out more heat just before a storm.

A fire hard to kindle indicates bad weather ahead.

Blacksmiths select a stormy day on which to prepare work requiring extra heat.

By Flowers: The perfume of flowers is more apparent just before a shower (when air is moist) than at any other time.

If the African marigold does not open its petals before 7:00 A.M., it will rain or thunder that day.

When cowslip (swamp plant or primrose) stalks are short, expect a dry summer.

By Horses: If horses stretch out their necks and sniff the air, rain will occur.

If horses startle more often than ordinary and are restless and uneasy or if they assemble in the corner of a field with their heads toward shelter, expect rain.

When horses and mules are very lively without apparent cause, look for chill. If they gather in tight huddles, rain and wind are on the way.

If you see a horse yawn, expect a shower of rain.

By Insects: If there are a lot of spiders in the fall, the winter will be bad.

Ants and spiders are very active when fair weather is on the way.

Ants move faster as the temperature rises. The cooler it gets, the slower they get.

Spiders make alteration in their web to suit the weather every twenty-four hours. When high wind or heavy rain threatens, a spider will be seen shortening the rope filaments that sustain the web structure. If a storm is to be unusually severe or of long duration, the ropes are strengthened as well as shortened. When you see the spider running out the slender filaments, it is certain that calm, fine weather has set in. When the spider sits quiet and dull in the middle of its web, rain is not far off. If it is active, however, and continues so during a shower, then it will be of brief duration and sunshine will follow.

Count the number of a cricket's chirps in fourteen seconds, add forty, and you will have the temperature.

Flies bite more often before a rainstorm. (Fish do also.)

If an ant builds its nest high, it will be a bad winter.

When butterflies gather in bunches in the air, winter is coming soon. If they migrate early, winter will be early.

It will rain if earthworms come to the surface of the ground.

The wooly worm tells of a bad winter if:

    1) he has a heavy coat;

    2) a lot of them are crawling about;

3) their movement seems unusually slow;

4) the black band on his back is wide—the more black than brown he is and/or the wider his black stripe, the worse the winter;

5) you see them crawling before the first frost.

By Katydids: When you hear the first katydid, plant corn.

The louder the katydids sing in August, the bigger the blizzards in December.

When katydids sing over wheat stubble, frost is six weeks away.

Three months after the first katydid begins hollerin', the first killing frost will come.

By the Moon: The number of days old the moon is at the first snow tells how many snows there will be that winter.

When the moon is near full, it is not likely to snow.

Look for twenty days of rain and wind if a new moon falls on Saturday.

Frost is more likely under a full or new moon. The moon makes tides in the atmosphere just as it makes tides in the ocean. The highest tides in the atmosphere come during the new and full moons. If the high moon tides are added to the effect of a high-pressure area, doesn't it seem reasonable that frost is more likely?

Most freezes occur between the full moon and the last quarter. When the moon is near full, it never storms.

If there is a ring around the moon, it will rain. Count the stars in the ring, and it will rain within that many days.

It will rain within three days if the horns of the moon point down.

By Plants: Winter will be bad if:

1) pine cones open early;

2) moss grows heavy on the trees;

3) leaves shed before they turn;

4) tree bark is heaviest on the north side;

5) carrots grow deeper;

6) trees are laden with green leaves late in fall;

7) the crop of holly and dogwood berries is heavy;

8) bark on trees is thicker;

9) onions grow more layers;

10) sweet potatoes have a tougher skin.

By Sheep: If old sheep turn their backs toward the wind and remain so for some time, wet and windy weather is coming.

If sheep gambol or fight or retire to shelter, it presages a change in weather.

Old sheep are said to eat greedily before a storm and sparingly before a thaw.

For Snow: A red sky at sunrise followed quickly by a change to lemon yellow means a storm followed by cold weather.

F

Count the number of ground fogs in August, and you will know the number of snows for the winter.

If a shivering cold feeling is caused by high humidity and not the cold itself, these shivers often foretell sizeable storms when the actual temperature may not even be far below freezing.

A shift in the wind can foretell snow.

A bright spot like a second sun appearing on the horizon to one side of the sun (most frequently observed at sunrise) indicates the approach of snow shoveling.

High, thin cirrus clouds (better known as mares' tails) run in advance of storms by a day or two.

Sound can be heard for long distances just before a storm.

A halo around the moon or sun indicates approaching snow.

Birds try to eat as much as they can before a storm.

Watch a jet airplane overhead. If the jet stream or trail fades quickly, the weather will hold fair. If it hangs in the sky and enlarges into wide bands across the sky, a change in the weather is near.

It's a sign of snow if the fire on the hearth makes a noise like a body walking on snow or tramping snow.

By Stars: When the stars begin to huddle, the earth will soon become a puddle.

When the sky seems very full of stars, expect rain or, in winter, frost.

By Tides: Showers occur more frequently at the turn of the tide.

If, during the absence of wind, the surface of the sea becomes agitated by long rolling swells, a gale may be expected.

If, after the first ebb of the tide, it flows again for a little while, a storm approaches.

By Trees: When the locust trees blossom, you can safely take off your long underwear.

When beechnuts are plentiful, expect a mild winter.

If the blooms of dogwood trees are full, expect a cold winter; when the blooms are light, expect a mild winter.

It will rain if leaves show their backs.

It will rain within three days if you see a tree with a black snake in it.

Some will say you can keep the rain from coming if you will stick pins in a locust tree.

By Weather: Lots of low, rolling thunder in the late fall means a bad winter.

If it snows crosslegged, it will be a deep one.

A late frost means a bad winter.

Two frosts and lots of rain mean cold weather is near.

A long, hot summer means a long, cold winter. The hotter the summer, the colder the winter.

It will rain the same time the next day if the sun shines while it rains.

If the sun sets with clouds, it will rain.

If it rains on Easter Sunday, it will rain every Sunday for seven weeks.

If it hasn't rained in a long time and it starts to rain before 7:00 A.M., it will quit before 11:00 A.M.

You can count on a mild winter if the first killing frost comes late. If it comes early, watch out.

A dry and cold March means a good harvest, and a wet March means a bad harvest.

If it thunders in January, there will be frost in May. If it warms up and storms and thunders in January, don't rush the garden season and put out tender plants in the month of May.

If it storms and thunders in the winter months, it will turn cold within twenty-four hours. Watch livestock, especially cattle. Even swine will carry what they can gather up to warm their beds.

If there be ice in November that will bear a duck, there'll be nothing thereafter but sleet and muck.

If you sometimes have an overwhelming urge to get out into the open, you could have the ability to anticipate earthquakes.

FORTUNE — Don't fold your hands and wait for a fortune to fall into your lap. Twenty men remain hopelessly poor waiting for a fortune while one is made rich by the longed-for transaction of the dried-up uncle or grandfather.

FOUNTAIN — If an indoor drinking fountain is desired outside and would be a handy device for the family, install a faucet upside down on an outside outlet.

FOUNTAIN OF YOUTH — Eat a lot of chicken livers.

FOXGLOVE — Did you know that digitalis, the heart stimulant, is made from the dried leaves of a plant commonly known as purple foxglove?

FRECKLES (TO REMOVE) — Mix lemon juice and buttermilk and apply.

Grapevine sap seems to help.

FREEZES — Most freezes occur between the full moon and the last quarter.

FROSTBITE — Gently warm the affected area. Do not rub the frostbitten skin and do not expose it to heat that is too hot because the numbed skin cannot feel the heat.

Drink a lot of hot liquids.

Do not smoke because it constricts blood vessels.

Dress warmly in layers and be sure to protect your head.

FRUIT ROLLS — These treats may not be all natural. Check them out. Some fruit bars get more than 50 percent of their calories from added sugar. Real fruit bars contain no added sugar.

F

FUMIGATE (HOME) — Burn some cedar branches in your fireplace. The smoke will make everything smell good.

FUNNEL — Make a temporary funnel for small things with an envelope by cutting off one corner.

FURNITURE (TO CLEAN) — Mix three pints of linseed oil with one pint of spirits of turpentine. Put on with a cloth. When the polish dries, rub with a clean, soft cloth.

FURNITURE (POLISH) — Make and bottle for future use. Mix one tablespoon turpentine, three tablespoons of linseed oil, and one quart of hot water. Apply to furniture. Dry at once with a soft cloth. Rub to polish. Or mix equal parts of vinegar and cooking oil boiled for ten minutes. Rub in until the surface is well polished.

FURNITURE (SCRATCHES) — Dissolve a teaspoon of instant coffee in a teaspoon of water and apply.

Fish-a-lex Attractor

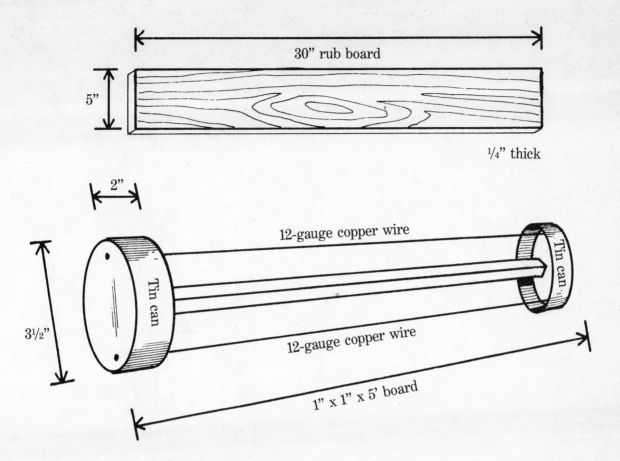

1. Use one 1" x 1" x 5' board.

2. Fasten this board to two tin cans (one on each end).

3. Cut two pieces of 12-gauge insulated copper wire, each five feet, three inches in length.

4. Fasten this 12-gauge wire on each side of the wood with tape.

5. Cut two holes in each tin can for bolts that will be used to fasten the wire to the can.

6. It does not matter how deep underwater this Fish Attractor is. Experiment with it at different depths. Hold the piece that is underwater. Rub a ¼" x 5" x 30" piece of wood edgewise across the top of the tin can for approximately thirty to forty-five seconds. Fish within a twenty-five- to thirty-foot radius should be attracted by this time.

Please let me know how this works for you.

Frymire Fish Finder and Attractor

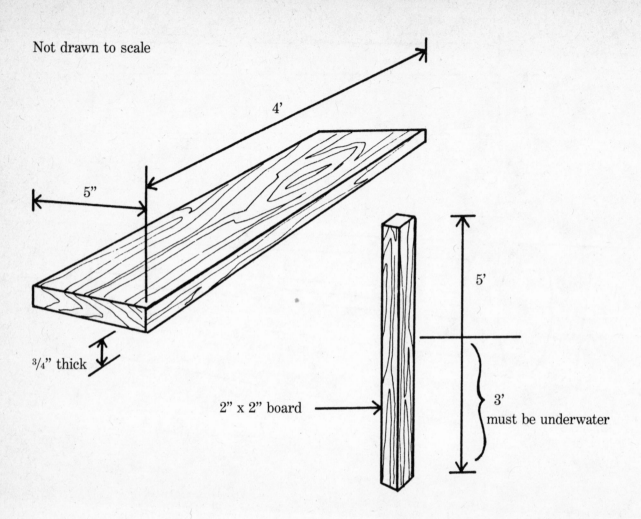

Not drawn to scale

4'

5"

³/₄" thick

5'

2" x 2" board

3' must be underwater

It makes very little difference what type of wood is used. You will need two pieces, one 2" x 2" x 5' and the other ³/₄" x 5" x 4'.

The most important thing to remember is that three feet of the 2" x 2" x 5' piece of wood must be underwater. This will require being in a boat in most cases. It would be best for Person 1 to hold the piece of wood that is in the water. Person 2 should rub the ³/₄" x 5" x 4' piece across the top for approximately thirty to forty-five seconds. Fish within a twenty-five- to thirty-foot radius should be attracted by this time.

Do not let the part that is underwater touch dirt.

Please let me know how this works for you. Eighty percent of the people who write after trying the fish attractor say that the invention works for them.

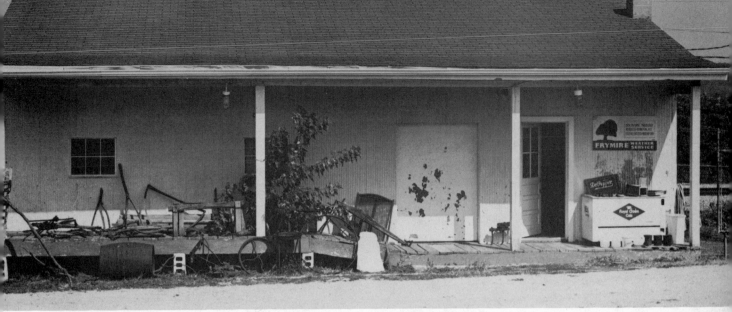

Frymire's Weather Service and Museum — Home Office

Horse-Drawn Wheat Binder

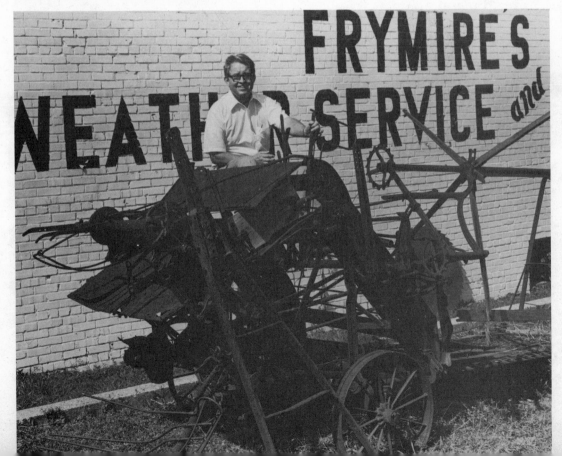

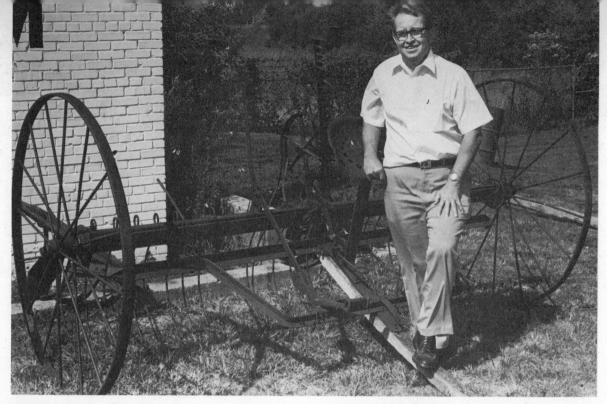

Horse-Drawn Hay Rake

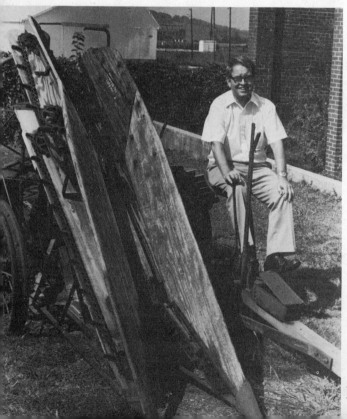

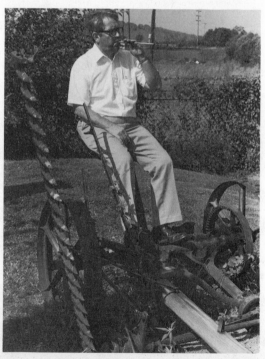

Horse-Drawn Mowing Machine

Horse-Drawn Corn Binder

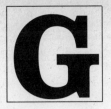

GALL BLADDER (PROBLEMS) — Start with one tablespoon of virgin olive oil and work up to one-quarter cup in grapefruit juice every morning. Do this for twenty days.

Mix one ounce of vegetable oil with four ounces of grapefruit juice. Do this for twenty-four days.

For three days drink apple juice. Do not eat or drink anything else. At the end of the second day and third day, drink one-half cup of olive oil with one-half cup of apple juice.

Some people advise taking one teaspoon of olive oil every twelve hours for five days.

Apply castor-oil packs for one hour twice daily for five days. Place packs over the lower area of the liver.

GALLS (HARNESS OR SADDLE) — Mix linseed oil with white lead. Apply with a brush. An airtight coating is formed to soothe the pain and assist nature.

GAME — To remove the fishy taste from game, peel a fresh lemon so as not to break the white inside skin. Put the lemon inside fresh fowl and keep it there for forty-eight hours, replacing it every twelve hours. All the fishy taste will be removed. A lemon prepared like this will remove unpleasant flavors from all meats and game.

GARDEN TIPS — Soil damage is our number-one problem. When we heal the soil, we will not have to heal man or animal.

Position garden stakes so the wind blows plants toward the supports, not away from them.

Growing squash or pumpkin vines among your corn will help keep out raccoons.

Rub seeds with sulphur and orange peelings before planting.

Spring planting should be done when the moon is waxing. The polarized light of the moon will bring faster growth.

Plant nasturtiums and marigolds in the garden to discourage nematodes and aphids.

Use an old curtain rod as a stake to support a plant. Pull up the rod's extension, and the two can grow together.

Do not plow closer than six feet to any fruit tree.

Pick cucumbers before they turn yellow, eggplant when it's glossy, zucchini when it's about six inches long.

G

Beans and cucumbers grow better when planted in conjunction with each other.

The rose bug or beetle should be killed by hand.

Seaweed meal and liquid seaweed are good for the soil.

Test your soil with garlic: if it grows like mad, your soil is rich.

Mulch your tomato vines, and place them around your peach and plum trees. This should get rid of insects.

Water vegetable and fruit trees with a solution of iron. They will grow to a very large size. This mixture, when used on flowers, will make them much brighter in color.

Never let fertilizer come in contact with roots until they have begun to grow.

It has been estimated that in a single year more than ten tons of dry earth per acre passes through the digestive system of earthworms and that in a field well populated with them one inch of topsoil will be created every five years. This being the case, it would be best not to apply a heavy application of chemical fertilizers and pesticides. If you do, a field can lose its earthworm population, which is important to keeping it in the state of health necessary to the production of nutritious crops.

If you wish to improve your soil, apply 250 pounds of kelp per acre. Also use seaweed meal and liquid seaweed extract.

Never prune a vine in frosty weather nor when frost is expected.

Use a good subsoiler on your land each year. It will help bring the soil back to life.

A dose of birth control pills dissolved in water is very good for tomato plants.

GARDEN TOOLS — To keep from losing your garden tools, paint them bright red. They will be much easier to spot.

GARLIC — Garlic has been used as medication by all ancient civilizations. Some say it is as important to our existence as air, earth, water, and fire. I don't think that I would go that far. Here are some of the things that people have discovered that garlic is good for: headaches, dizziness, infections, wound healing, cancer, aging, arthritis, worms, indigestion, gas pains, diarrhea, skin diseases, fungus, psoriasis, acne, TB, bronchitis, colds, pneumonia, influenza, diphtheria, cholera, typhoid, heart problems, high blood pressure, and clotting.

Place a little garlic near your fruit trees to ward off certain insects or bugs. Human hair (obtained from your local barber) should be placed near trees and the garden to help in controlling bugs, insects, and deer.

Garlic has stimulant and antiseptic qualities good for diarrhea, low blood pressure, and earache.

Some say that germs cannot live in the presence of garlic.

Remember, if you are afraid of garlic breath, all you need to do is chew parsley chlorophyl tablets.

If your digestion can't cope with fresh garlic, take capsules of garlic and parsley oils.

GAS — Steep one-quarter teaspoon of powdered ginger in a cup of hot water for five minutes. Drink as needed.

Take anise seeds.

GEESE — Be sure to feed your geese raw potatoes if you expect to eat them. They will have a much better flavor. Don't forget that in old geese, the bills and feet are red. In young ones, they are yellow.

GINSENG — Ginseng will grow best in a dark and damp place. It usually takes five or six years for ginseng to mature. You can tell if it is ripe because of its red seeds. You make the tea out of the roots.

Ginseng (pronounced jin-seng in most places but simply 'sang in other parts) looks very much like any other root to the untrained eye: brown, gnarled and about as large as a little finger. It is sometimes called man-root and man-essence. It is also sometimes called holy herb and wonder-of-the-world. One pound of marketable dried ginseng means finding and digging, with a short-handled mattock, two hundred fresh roots, three and one-half pounds' worth. A good ginseng worker can make about $150 for eighteen hours of work. Ginseng usually grows on the north or west side of hardwood forests. After six or seven years of growing, the plant reaches a height of two feet or so and has reached maturity. Its top is filled with bright berries that 'sang hunters look for on their autumn forays. Starting in 1977, ginseng became an endangered plant species, and hunters are now required to replant the berries. The average ginseng root seldom weighs as much as two ounces. Someone once told me that the record weight for one wild ginseng root was one pound, four ounces.

GLASSWARE — When glassware develops nicks on the edges, rub them smooth again with fine sandpaper.

To prevent glassware from cracking in hot water, slip it into the water sideways.

GOLD CHAINS (TO CLEAN) — Wash them in soap suds and rinse in diluted alcohol. Lay in a box of dry cedar sawdust.

GOLDENROD — Goldenrod roots are good for checking your bowels. If you have bowel trouble, just dig the roots, wash them, and chew.

GOLDENSEAL — Goldenseal is a short, hardy plant with greenish white blossoms. Make a tea out of it or eat it dry. The tea makes a good eyewash. If you are sore, beat up some goldenseal with mutton tallow or soot from an old woodstove. This makes an excellent salve for humans or animals.

GOUT (CURE) — Mix hot vinegar and salt together. Be sure the salt dissolves. Rub in with your hand and dry the foot. Rub in for at least fifteen minutes each time. Do this four times a day for five days, then twice a day for five days, then once a day for five days.

Eat twenty fresh cherries a day for twenty days, then ten a day thereafter. Canned cherries work for some people. There are some people who say take one tablespoon of cherry concentrate three times a day.

GREENS — Do not soak fresh vegetables or salad greens in water for any great length of time. Soaking dissolves the minerals and reduces the vitamin content.

Greens such as collard, mustard, turnip, and kale also have a fair share of calcium. Broccoli is also good.

GROUNDHOG — To get rid of groundhogs, roll up some Juicy Fruit gum and stick it in their burrows.

Gout (Big Toe) Pain Reliever or Gout Zapper

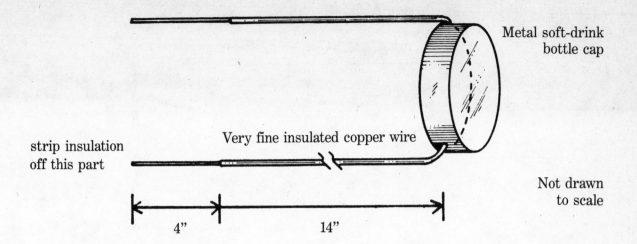

strip insulation off this part

Very fine insulated copper wire

Metal soft-drink bottle cap

Not drawn to scale

4" 14"

1. Assemble the following materials: one metal soft-drink bottle cap and two eighteen-inch pieces of very fine insulated copper wire.

2. On one end of each wire, strip off four inches of the insulation.

3. On the other end of each wire, strip off one-quarter inch of the insulation.

4. Close to the edge of the bottle cap, bore two holes the size of the copper wire.

5. Place one quarter-inch piece of copper wire through the hole in the bottle cap and solder. Then place the other one-quarter-inch piece of copper wire through the other hole and solder.

6. Wrap each four-inch end of the copper wire around the big toe.

7. Soak a 1" x 18" piece of cloth in warm castor oil and gently wring it out.

8. Wrap this cloth around the big toe, around which the copper wire is wrapped.

9. Hold the bottle cap with one hand. Then take a wooden ruler with the other hand and rub it across the top of the cap for two minutes. Rest for five minutes and repeat.

10. Do this five times a day for three days.

11. Soak some coarse brown paper in apple-cider vinegar. Apply this around the big toe between treatments.

12. Drink at least sixteen ounces of water after each treatment.

*Green-Thumbs—Write Dick with
ten ways you make your garden grow.*

1. _____

2. _____

3. _____

4. _____

5. _____

6. _____

7. _____

8. _____

9. _____

10. _____

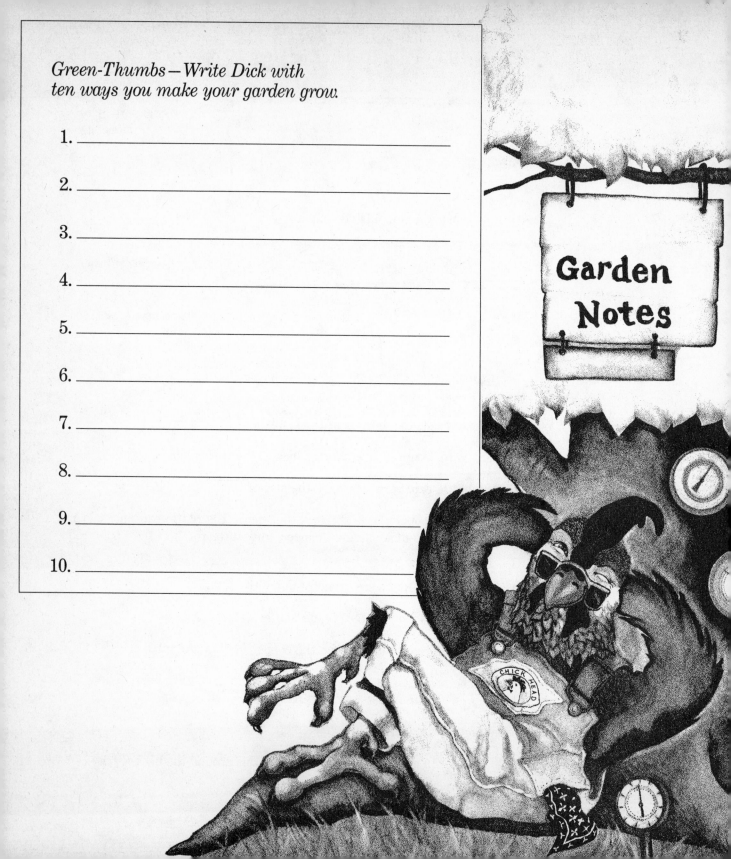

Garden
Notes

CHICK HEAD

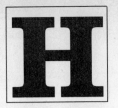

HAIR — Healthy, Attractive Hair, To Maintain: Massage the scalp with five drops of castor oil.

Massage the scalp twice a week with Listerine.

Wear a scarf or hat when you are in the sun to keep the hair soft and shiny.

Allow your hair to dry naturally, patting it dry rather than rubbing it.

To increase hair luster, let a mixture of one pint of boiling water and two tablespoons of dried rosemary soak for three hours. Then massage the head with it.

Always rinse your hair after exposure to chlorine.

Be sure to get plenty of vitamins A and C and iodine to prevent dryness.

Adequate copper intake prevents defects in pigmentation of the hair.

Hair Loss, To Prevent: Wet the hair two times a week with milk or a weak solution of salt water.

Take zinc and B-complex vitamins.

Rub the fingernails of your right hand across the fingernails of your left hand. Do this three times a day for five minutes each time.

Mix one tablespoon of honey with one-quarter cup of onion juice. Massage the scalp twice a day for five minutes each time.

An hour before going to bed, rub a fresh-cut clove of garlic on the hairless area. Wait one hour and then massage the scalp with olive oil.

Stand on your head for five minutes each day. (Note: Do not do this if you have low or high blood pressure.)

Rub a mixture of one jigger of vodka and one-half teaspoon of cayenne pepper on the scalp.

Hair, Washing and Rinsing: If you can't actually wash your hair, you can dry clean it. Sprinkle a piece of cheesecloth with cologne, cover a brush with the cloth, and brush your hair thoroughly. Your hair will look and smell clean.

A good rinse for the hair is four tablespoons of vinegar per half-gallon of water.

To make your hair shine, whip two egg yolks and apply into freshly shampooed, towel-dried hair. Let the treatment sit for five minutes, then rinse it off.

H

Hair, To Remove Unwanted: Eat raw and cooked vegetables and foods high in iodine, such as potato peelings and seafood.

HANDS (BROWN SPOTS) — Mix two tablespoons of sulphur with one-half cup of milk. Let the sulphur settle to the bottom. After three hours rub the milk part on the brown spots twice a day for ten days, then once a day.

HANDS (CLEANER) — After lathering up with soap, sprinkle a little salt or sugar on your hands. The granules help scrub off the grease and grime.

Lightly coat your hands with liquid soap before doing mechanical, gardening, or other heavy work. They will then clean rather easily.

Remove tar from your hands by rubbing them with the outside of a fresh orange or lemon peel and wiping them dry at once. Wash the hands in clear water and wipe lightly. While they are still moist, strike a match and shut your hands around it so as to catch the smoke. Then the stain will disappear.

Washing with a salt-and-lemon mixture will remove stains from the hands.

Ground mustard mixed with a little water is an excellent agent for cleansing the hands after handling odorous substances.

Remove walnut stains from the hands by rubbing with apple or pear slices or with the juice of ripe tomatoes.

If everything else fails, wash the hands in horseradish and milk.

HANDS (PERSPIRING) — Mix club moss in the water when you wash your hands.

HANDS (ROUGH) — Excessive use of salt will cause rough hands.

Chapped hands are liable to absorb poisonous matter into your system.

HANDS (SOFT) — Fill a bucket half full of fine sand and soap suds and water as hot as you can stand. Wash your hands for five minutes with this mixture, washing and rubbing them in the sand. Rinse in warm water and dry. Next rub the hands with cornmeal. Finish the job by rubbing them with hog lard (about one teaspoon).

Mix lemon juice and glycerine together. Rub into hands well.

HANDSHAKE — The handshake wasn't always a sign of friendship. It began as a way to tell if a weapon was being carried.

HANGOVER — Drink plenty of water and fruit juices. Lay off the coffee.

Drink a glass of water to which one-eighth of a teaspoon of cayenne pepper has been added.

Massage your thumbs just below the knuckles.

Every minute for five minutes, eat one tablespoon of honey. Repeat one-half hour later.

Rub one-quarter of a lemon on each armpit.

HARVEST DRINK — Mix five gallons of water, one-half gallon of molasses, one quart of vinegar, and two ounces of powdered ginger. This drink will give you a lift.

HEAD — A clean head prevents contagious diseases. Wash your head every day.

HEAD NOISE — Place a heating pad on your feet and hands.

Place a large brown paper sack over your head; breathe in and out fifteen or twenty times. Do this three times daily.

Head noise could be caused by using too many aspirin or other drugs.

Mix one tablespoon of vinegar, one tablespoon of honey, and six to eight ounces of water. Take three times daily, preferably at mealtime.

HEADACHE REMEDIES — **Twenty-one Causes of Headaches:**

Allergy	Exertion	Sinus infection
Aneurysm	Eye strain	Temporal acteritis
Arthritis	Fever	Temporo-mandibular joint syndrome
Caffeine withdrawal	Hangover	Tension
Classic migraine	Hunger	Tic douloureux
Common migraine	Hypertension	Trauma
Cluster headache	Menstruation	Tumor

Take a cloth or towel and soak it in ice water. Wring it out. Go into a dark, cool room and lie down, putting the towel or cloth on your forehead. Within fifteen minutes, you should get relief. In thirty minutes, you should be asleep.

This very simple exercise should prevent or cure headaches in 75 percent of cases. It is also good for improving eyesight in 10 percent of cases. It does not seem to help much when your headache is caused by high blood pressure. First, sit erect with your neck stretched. Bend the head back four times, then forward four times. Move to the left and to the right sides four times each. Next circle the head each way four times. Repeat the left-right movement and the circling. Don't rush—take your time while doing this exercise. The headache should be much better or cured. At the end of four months of doing this exercise regularly, twice a day, your eyesight should be much improved.

Take a brisk twenty-minute walk each morning and evening.

If the headache is caused by excessive reading, slowly sip a cup of fresh orange juice. Some say this relieves headaches in minutes.

Rub the second joint of each thumb, alternately for five times, two minutes each time.

Take one teaspoon of honey with one-half teaspoon of garlic juice.

One woman reports that immersing her hands in hot water cures her headaches.

Another woman reports that she rubs the back of her neck downward about three times a second for thirty seconds, cupping her hand. This cures her headaches.

You can make a headache remedy by making a tea of one-half teaspoon each of peppermint and skullcap. You can also take three or four calcium or dolomite tablets with this tea.

Drink two tablespoons of brewer's yeast each morning in a glass of juice.

Place your hands over the area where the headache is located.

Sniff some oxygen.

Many people suffer from a combination of headache and cold feet. To treat this ailment, they should plunge the feet into cold water every morning and use the flesh brush every night. This treatment should relieve both ailments.

Always eat a high-fiber diet.

Drink at least eight glasses of water per day.

Make sassafras tea as follows: Dig sassafras roots. Then take the white off the roots and discard. Take the remainder (which should be red in color) and cut into chips. Put the chips in a quart or two-quart pan and cover with water. Boil until the water becomes a deep reddish orange color. Then mix equal parts of sassafras tea and pure lemon juice from fresh lemons. Reheat this mixture and do not add any sweeteners. Drink a large hot cup.

The best way to avoid a hangover headache (other than not drinking) is to eat fatty foods and drink milk before indulging.

Concentrate on making your hands feel warm. This concentration will increase blood flow to the hands, thus relieving the headache.

After going to bed, sleep without the pillow.

Apply a bag of hot cornmeal to your head.

Spin around until you are dizzy.

Heat some mint and vinegar, then breathe the vapors.

Rub lemon rinds on your forehead and temples. Then place the rinds on your forehead, securing them with a scarf or bandage. Leave on for one hour.

Press your thumb against the roof of your mouth. Every so often, move your thumb to another section of the roof of the mouth.

Place both feet in ankle-deep ice water. Move them around in a leisurely manner for four minutes or for as long as it takes your feet to start feeling warm. When that happens, take them out and go directly to bed. Cover up, relax, and in no time there will be no more headache.

Eat strawberries. They contain organic salicylates, which are the active ingredient in aspirin.

Drink hounds-tongue and wild peppermint tea.

Migraine headaches: Nineteen foods to avoid if you suffer from migraines:

Aged meat	Nuts	Processed meats
Anchovies	Onions	Raisins
Avocados	Papayas	Raspberries
Bananas	Pickled herring	Sour cream
Canned figs	Plums	Yogurt
Chocolate		

Hot fresh bread or rolls (safe to eat after cooling)
Ripened cheeses (e.g., Stilton, Brie, Cheddar)
Seeds (sesame, sunflower, pumpkin)

Migraines may be cured by changing your pattern of living. Avoid eating aged cheese. Avoid chocolate and alcohol and reduce your coffee consumption. Do not get overweight or skip meals, not even a single meal. Reduce your weight if you are overweight, but eating regular meals is very important. Get up at the same time every day. Do not smoke excessively.

If you suffer from migraine headaches, do not cook in aluminum pots and pans.

Dipping cabbage leaves into hot water until they are soft, then applying them to the forehead and the back of the neck can relieve migraine headache pain.

Another migraine treatment is to boil two Spanish onions. Eat one and mash the other, placing the resulting paste on your forehead.

Take an enema with the following mixture: two teaspoons of salt, one teaspoon of soda, and one gallon of water at body temperature. Rinse with one and one-half quarts of water containing one tablespoon of Glyco-Thymoline.

Apply pressure to the palm of one hand with the thumb of the other hand. Then reverse the order. Keep up the pressure for five minutes on each hand.

The minute you feel a migraine coming on, take one tablespoon of honey. If the pain is not gone one-half hour later, take another tablespoon of honey and drink three glasses of water.

Sick headache: Soak some coarse brown paper in vinegar and place it on the forehead. If the eyelids are gently bathed in cool water, the pain in the head will subside.

A sick headache can often be greatly relieved and sometimes entirely cured by applying a mustard plaster at the base of the neck. The plaster should not be kept on for more than fifteen minutes.

A sick headache can be relieved by filling a tumbler full of finely crushed ice, lemon juice, and one teaspoon of white sugar. Mix well, and eat very slowly.

Sinus headache: Apply poultices of either raw grated onion or horseradish to the nape of the neck and the soles of the feet.

Sniff a little horseradish juice when you have a sinus headache.

H

Violent Headache: Put your feet in ankle-deep hot water. Leave them until the water starts to cool.

Acute violent headaches may be relieved by mixing one cup of ice with one-half cup of salt. Tie this mixture in a small linen cloth to make a pad. Place this close to the seat of pain.

Old-timers used to say that cases of extreme headache could be cured in a half-hour if the person would take a teaspoon of finely powdered charcoal in half a tumbler of water. They said this provided an innocent yet powerful alkali.

If you are suffering from a nervous headache, wash your hair in weak soda water. You should be almost wholly cured in ten minutes by this simple remedy. Be sure to dry the head thoroughly afterward.

Avoid drafts of air for a little while. Some find it the greatest relief in cases of "rare cold," with the cold symptoms leaving the eyes and nose entirely after one thorough washing of the hair.

HEALTH (HINTS) — Secrets of Good Health:
1) Always keep warm.
2) Eat regularly and slowly.
3) Maintain regular bodily habits.
4) Keep clear skin.
5) Get plenty of sleep.
6) Keep cheerful company.
7) Keep out of debt.
8) Don't set your mind on things you don't need.
9) Mind your business, and subdue curiosity.

America is the most fed and the worst nourished nation on earth. We are suffering from biological blight. We are facing metabolic disaster. We are a nation of sick people.

According to the Bible, God created man in his own image—a perfect being. After creation, man was placed in a garden where fruits, berries, edible leaves, roots, and honey were provided as his food. They were all acid in reaction and rich in minerals. Thus, the body that was designed for this sort of food has been subjected to the pressures of an utterly different environment in our time, but it still contains within itself the ability to adjust itself if we would only follow the original plan for daily food intake.

Check with a healthy person to see why he or she is healthy.

Always eat a light supper, never later than 6:00 P.M. For that in-between-meals snack, try some dried raisins, which should satisfy your craving for sweets. You will be getting a carbohydrate pickup from their natural sugar. Fructose, refined white sugar, contains sucrose. Raisins contain these minerals: iron, calcium, sodium, phosphorus, potassium, and magnesium. They also have some of the B-vitamins and, if you eat a whole cup, thirty-two units of vitamin A. Never eat sticky raisins.

Always rise in the morning the moment you awaken.

If you have high blood pressure, try viewing fish in an aquarium.

We need to turn to foods that do not come out of a factory. Eat more fruits, berries, edible leaves and roots, and honey. Live more out of the garden, the orchard, and the ocean. The apple-cider-vinegar cruet needs to be returned to the table, as does the honey receptacle.

Eat two oranges every morning before breakfast through the spring season, and you will need no medicine during the rest of the year.

Many of the potato's most valuable vitamins and minerals are in the skin itself. Don't waste it — eat it!

Liver and lung complaints benefit greatly from your eating onions, either cooked or raw. Even colds yield to this treatment. Eat onions regularly. Boil the juice of onions to a syrup and take this as a medicine. But eating boiled, roasted, or fried onions is even better for you.

Always put a green leaf under your hat while you work outside in hot weather.

Charcoal and honey, mixed together and used as a dentifrice, will whiten teeth.

If you do a lot of brain work, you will need to sleep more.

If you are bent over, walk with your hands behind you.

A good laugh is worth a hundred groans.

File the top of an ingrown toenail very thin and place cotton under the ingrown part.

If you will cut the hind legs of your chair a little shorter than the front ones, the fatigue of sitting will be lessened and your spine will be in a better position.

If you are wakeful at night, get up, walk about the room, and then take fifteen deep breaths.

Do not let the temperature in your home go above seventy degrees.

If you get your clothes wet, leave them on till they dry. If you do this, you will not have a cold.

Children should be encouraged to eat without drinking so that they may be led to moisten their food with saliva, thus preparing themselves to have good digestion.

Take or eat five tablespoons of dried coconut meat daily if you are high strung.

Mix one cup of fresh blackberries, three tablespoons of sugar, and five tablespoons of whiskey. Take one tablespoon every hour until you are well.

Any room that is too warm and dry for window plants is unfit to live in.

Acid of the right kind, such as apple-cider vinegar, may destroy germs and viruses in the intestine.

In the morning, thirty minutes before breakfast, take the juice of one lemon in a goblet of water. This will make your system ready for the day ahead.

H

People in the north need to eat more apples, grapes, cranberries, leafy root vegetables, berries, honey, nuts, fish, game, and poultry. It wouldn't hurt to take kelp tablets, either.

HEART (PAIN) — Eat alfalfa sprouts every day.

Drink peppermint tea.

Sip a little champagne or dry white wine daily.

Massage the pads at the base of the last two fingers on the left hand or massage the left foot under the third, fourth, and fifth toes. This can relieve heart pain within seconds.

Eat the red part of red roses raw.

HEART (TO STRENGTHEN) — Eat wheat germ every day.

Eat a lot of garlic.

HEART (WEAK) — Burn the roots of a wild grapevine into a black ash. Mix one teaspoon of this black ash with one-half cup of water and drink. You will find this works as well as any diuretic.

HEARTBURN — Eat a slice of raw potato.

Eat a raw carrot.

Eat two peach-pit kernels once a day for four days.

Never lie down when you have heartburn.

Eat six almonds, chewing each one thirty times.

Grate a raw potato and squeeze out all of the juice. Add twice the amount of warm water and drink.

Add the juice of one-half lemon and one-half teaspoon of salt to a cup of warm water and drink.

HEATING PAD — Here's how to get along without a rubber hot water bottle. Put a small bag of salt into a skillet and heat. Then wrap the bag in closely woven cloth. It will hold its heat for a long time.

HEMORRHOIDS — Increase your fiber and fluid intake.

Eat four almonds a day.

Insert a peeled clove of garlic in the rectum right after a bowel movement.

Cut a peeled raw potato in the shape of a suppository and insert it in the rectum.

Chop a handful of cranberries finely. Wrap a tablespoon or so in a piece of cheesecloth and tuck into the rectal area. Apply a new compress every hour.

Crush a handful of soybeans and apply as a compress.

HENS — Hens that lay commercial eggs are cooped up where they cannot move and have seldom, if ever, seen a rooster, let alone been caught by one. This poses a question: How can an unhappy hen lay a good egg?

HERBS — In the spring, always gather enough roots and herbs to do you until the next spring.

Many have written to say that boneset and pennyroyal are the best medicinal herbs.

HERNIA — Soak a cloth in castor oil and apply it to the hernia area. Place a warm towel over this cloth. Leave on for thirty minutes.

Apply a castor-oil pack to the abdomen for a hiatal hernia.

Eat one-third of a medium-sized raw potato.

HERPES — Apply vitamin-E oil.

Apply plain yogurt to the affected area and after a few minutes wash it off. Now repeat the process with raw honey.

HICCUPS — Swallow a teaspoon of fresh onion juice.

Gently inhale a little pepper, just enough to make you sneeze.

Place an ice cube right below the Adam's apple and count to one hundred.

Take a hot bath.

Try breathing into a brown paper bag.

Plug your ears while you drink some water.

Splash some cold water on the back of your neck.

Mix one teaspoon of sugar with one teaspoon of vinegar. Take as needed.

Eat a teaspoon of peanut butter.

Eating plum jelly will cure severe cases of hiccups.

Chew some dill seed.

Take a glass of water and put a towel over the glass. Take eight to ten sips of water through the towel.

Suck on a wedge of lemon.

Drink one-half ounce of cider vinegar. Take it straight all at once.

Try this remedy, which has been reported always to work: Put a knife in a glass of water with the blade in the water and the handle up. Press the handle of the knife against your temple. Slowly drink the water. That should stop your hiccups.

H

HIVES — Mix one teaspoon of cream of tartar with six ounces of water and drink.

For itching associated with hives, take a hot bath with soda. Use two and one-half cups of soda in a large tub.

Apply cool buttermilk to hives.

Mix one tablespoon of cider vinegar, one tablespoon of local honey, and eight ounces of water. Sip with each meal.

Use no products that contain caffeine.

HOARSENESS — Bake a lemon for twenty minutes in a moderate oven. Dig out the insides, sweeten with molasses, and eat.

Eat some horseradish.

For hoarseness due to a cold, beat the white of one egg, add the juice of one lemon, and sweeten with sugar. Take a teaspoon as needed.

HOLE (DIG) — Dig a hole on the new of the moon (growing moon, increasing in size), and you will have dirt to throw away if you try to fill it up. Dig it on the old of the moon (day after the full moon, decreasing in size), and you will not have enough dirt to fill it back up.

Dig a post hole during the growing of the moon and put a post in it. It'll be loose all the time and never settle. Dig the same hole on the old of the moon, just the same size, and sink your post. It will settle tight.

HOLE (IN SCREEN) — Plug a small hole in a window screen with a drop of model airplane glue.

HOME (BEFORE BUYING) — Before buying your dream home, do this: Jump up and down in the center of the room. If the house seems to shake apart, don't buy it.

HONEY — Applied externally, honey is nourishing and soothing to the skin. Internally, honey is a quick source of energy and a mild sedative.

If honey goes to sugar, heat it in a pan or place it in a microwave oven.

Honey is used in the treatment of many disorders. It has been used to treat asthma, hay fever, allergies, digestive problems, hemorrhoids, arthritis, cuts and wounds, bad complexions, and coughs and colds. You should always try to use raw, unprocessed honey.

Never give honey to a child less than one year old.

HOOSIER — The word hoosier got started, according to the story told by my very reliable cousin Allen Hamilton, many years ago in Battletown, Kentucky. It seems that there was much feuding between the Greers and the Bennetts of Kentucky and the Fosters and Jacobses of Indiana. During one big fight, the Greers and the Bennetts cut off the ears of the Fosters and the Jacobses. After the Fosters and Jacobses had crossed the river to get back into Indiana, there was a rather large number of ears in a pile. The Kentucky boys got to asking "Who's ear is that?" Since that time, the question has evolved into "Hoosier."

HORSE (BALKY) — Buckle a strap to the horse's foreleg close to his breast. Throw the other end over his shoulder, then buckle it near his hoof so that it is nearly touching his belly. Leave him this way for a while so that his mind can be diverted from the cause that stopped him.

You can also try just tying the horse where he stops. Leave him standing there for about four hours. Then he should be glad to go.

When your horse balks, try taking him from the carriage and whirling him around till he is giddy. Keep him in the smallest circle possible, and don't let him step out. It takes two men to do this. One dose should cure, and two doses are sure to do so.

HOT FLASHES — Eat a cucumber a day.

HORSERADISH — This is good for treating sinusitis, stimulating the appetite, and aiding in digestion. You can prepare your own by grating a fresh horseradish root. Then mix it with an equal amount of lemon juice. You can also buy this already prepared at the grocery store.

HOUSEHOLD HINTS — For a high polish on furniture, go over the entire surface with a cloth dampened with equal parts of raw linseed oil and turpentine. Wipe off the excess oil with a cloth and polish with a dry woolen cloth.

To remove water stains on antique furniture, rub mayonnaise into the grain, then polish with a soft cloth.

Bottle this homemade solution, then use it as needed to remove sticky fingerprints from furniture. Add three tablespoons of linseed oil and one tablespoon of turpentine to one quart of hot water. Mix well. Let cool. Wring a soft cloth out in this solution and apply to furniture. Dry at once with a soft cloth. Rub to a polish.

Once or twice a year give wooden furniture a bath in the following way: Make a light lather out of mild soap and lukewarm water. Wring a soft cloth out in this lather. Wash a small area at a time. Then, before you go farther, rinse with a cloth wrung out in clear lukewarm water. Dry at once with another soft cloth. Then keep going with the same routine, but start just within the clean area each time. Apply furniture wax or polish according to the manufacturer's directions when you are finished with the bath.

Varnished surfaces can usually be cleaned nicely with a cloth dipped in cool, weak tea. That's right! — cool, weak tea.

To polish antiques or old pieces, use a mixture of two parts turpentine to one part of linseed oil or equal parts of turpentine, linseed oil, and vinegar. Apply with a soft cloth and rub. Polish with a dry cloth.

To make scratches in mahogany "invisible," dye them with iodine. The same idea works well on other dark woods. Rub light scratches with the cut surface of walnut meat or Brazil-nut meat.

To remove alcohol stains from furniture, go over the spot with a cloth dampened in lemon oil, using a circular motion. Then dip the cloth in powdered rottenstone, just enough to soil it. Gently rub powder on the stain. Wipe off the surface with another cloth moistened with lemon oil. Dry and polish with a soft, clean cloth. If necessary, repeat the treatment.

Eradicate white spots on mahogany furniture by spreading a thick coat of Vaseline over the spots and letting it stand for forty-eight hours before wiping it off.

Wicker furniture should be cleaned by scrubbing it with a stiff brush moistened with warm salt water. Salt keeps the wicker from turning yellow.

Don't shake your dust-mop out the window if you want your neighbors to love you. Tie a big paper bag around the mop head and shake vigorously. Then throw the bag and dust away.

To brighten a rug, sprinkle salt over it before using the vacuum cleaner. This makes it easier to remove soot.

Very tiny scratches on waxed woodwork surfaces can be concealed by rubbing them with wax.

White furniture can be cleaned by dissolving baking soda in warm water and applying the solution to the furniture with a soft cloth. Use a teaspoon of the solution to a pint of water.

Wipe piano keys with a cloth slightly dampened in denatured alcohol. Wipe dry with a soft cloth. (Note: Never use soap on the keys. Soap stains ivory.)

The piano may be a large instrument, but it is a very delicate one. So don't try to clean the inside. Leave this to the expert who "voices" it at regular intervals.

Never use furniture polish or oil on the case of your piano. Dust with soft, untreated cloth.

An easy and economical way to clean copper is to dip half a lemon in salt and rub the object. Rinse in hot water and polish with a soft cloth.

When your arms are loaded with grocery bags and boxes, a small shelf on a bracket beside the back door will provide a place for unloading and give you a chance to get at keys and the door knob. Such a shelf will also hold milk and other deliveries out of the reach of neighborhood dogs and cats.

Press a dab of white toothpaste into nail and tack holes left when you take down pictures and posters. Let the paste dry, paint over it, and presto! The ugly holes are gone.

Wash furniture with warm soap suds. Quickly wipe it dry, then rub it with an oily cloth.

Bring brightness to that old faded oil painting by gently wiping the surface with a fresh-cut onion.

Nail a mousetrap on the wall in the cellar or shed to hold work gloves, a cap, instruction charts, etc. It makes a special place for easily mislaid belongings.

A warm knife will easily smooth icing on a cake.

Grained wood should be washed with cold tea.

To purify damp rooms and closets, place a bucket or tray of quicklime in damp places generating mildew. Renew the quicklime from time to time.

If you love your fine china, put paper doilies between plates and saucers when stacking them to prevent scratches. Never, never hang cups by the handles or stack them. Set them in a row instead.

Porcelain is easily cleaned with salt sprinkled on a flannel cloth.

Clean your candles with a cloth dampened in alcohol.

Wash all varnished wood with tea. It requires very little rubbing, as the tea acts as a strong detergent, cleansing the paint of its impurities and making the varnish shine like new. Tea also washes windowpanes and mirrors much better than soap and water. But it will not do to wash unvarnished paint with it.

Margarine, when applied and rubbed persistently, will loosen tar marks on your vinyl floors. When it comes to heel marks, try baking soda and water.

Add a tablespoon of molasses to stove blacking to make it adhere better and retain its polish longer.

To keep your stovetop smooth, roll up a piece of flannel and dip it in fine sand. Rub the stove after cooking.

Sparkling car windows are possible with a mixture of one-half cup of cornstarch and two quarts of warm water applied to the area. Wipe dry with an absorbent cloth.

A thimble over·the ends of your curtain rods will stop snags in the curtains.

Stop static shock in carpeting by mixing one part of liquid fabric softener and five parts of water in a mist bottle and spraying the mixture over the carpet.

Pecans, when rubbed onto furniture scratches, will darken the damaged area so that it matches the surrounding wood.

Water rings on furniture can be removed with white toothpaste and a damp cloth. Remember to polish with furniture polish afterward.

Cover the bottom of an electric frying pan with an ammonia-soaked cloth. Then place the skillet in a plastic bag, tie it shut, and let it stand overnight. Grease and stains will then come off easily.

To make a cobweb duster, roll up a newspaper, place a rubber band over the center of the roll, and snip the ends of the paper.

Try colorless lacquer on brass and copper to protect their surfaces from corrosion.

H

A ventilating fan in the kitchen or bath should be turned on only long enough to accomplish its job. Let it run unnoticed and a houseful of hot or cold air can be drawn out very quickly.

Don't burn colored comic sheets in a grill or fireplace. The lead in the ink goes into the food and air. Offset printing presents no hazard, but when in doubt, don't.

Do you have a small crack in your wood stove that permits small amounts of smoke to escape? If so, wood ashes and common salt, made compact with water, will stop the crack.

Remove all window screens in winter to get maximum solar warmth, then clean the glass of dust and grime.

Attached garages require less heat than house interiors do. A forty-degree-Fahrenheit temperature is adequate and better for your car.

To loosen a stiff door lock, lubricate the key by rubbing it with soap.

Oil your fan by getting a flexible drinking straw and placing it over the oil hole. Squirt the oil into the other end of the straw.

Dried corncobs make good scrubbers for especially dirty jobs.

Dried coffee grounds make a good filling for a pin cushion.

Use straight pins to hold pictures. Drive them into the wall at a forty-five-degree angle. Sewing machine needles work well, too, and they are stronger. They both leave a much smaller hole than a nail.

Remove paper stuck to any wood by first allowing a few drops of oil to soak into it and then rubbing gently with a clean cloth.

Make your own treated dusters this way: Dip eighteen-inch cheesecloth squares in a solution of two cups of hot water and one-quarter cup of lemon oil. Squeeze out excess liquid and dry.

A safe way to gather up small pieces of broken glass is to pat them up with a dampened absorbent cloth.

Clean and shine mirrors at the same time by adding a little borax to the water used for washing them. Another way to brighten mirrors is to rub them with a cloth dampened with a little alcohol.

Remove paint splashes from windows and mirrors by washing them with turpentine, ammonia, or hot vinegar. Never use a razor as it may scratch the glass.

Picture glass is best cleaned with a cloth wrung out in hot water and dipped in alcohol. Polish it once with a chamois cloth until it is dry and glossy.

Give glazed wall tiles the sparkle of newness by wiping them with a sponge dipped in ammonia and water.

You can usually do away with light scratches on shellacked, varnished, or waxed floors with a solution containing equal parts of turpentine, boiled linseed oil, and white vinegar.

White spots on your shellacked floors (usually due to spilled water) can easily be removed with a cloth moistened with equal parts of denatured alcohol and turpentine.

This sounds silly, but it works! Stale, soft chunks of bread, rubbed over wallpaper in even vertical strokes, "erase" the soiled spots—even very visible fingerprints.

Baking soda and vinegar can clean your toilet bowl.

Salt can be used on oven spills. Wet the cooled oven, then apply a thin layer of salt. Let it stand a few minutes and wipe away.

To remove iron rust from white goods, use sour milk.

Freezing moist steel-wool pads in plastic freezer bags prevents rusting.

To remove rust from the corners of cake tins that have not been in use for a long time, dip a raw potato in cleaning powder and scour with it.

To remove rusty screws, pour a little kerosene over them, and the rust will give way after they soak for a short time.

Place aluminum foil, shiny-side up, between the ironing board and the cover pad. It reflects heat and cuts down on ironing time.

HUNTERS — Wash your clothes with Arm & Hammer baking soda to mask any scents that might tip off your prey.

HYDRANGEAS — Hydrangeas' colors reflect the pH of the soil. A pink color denotes an alkaline condition; a blue flower, acid soil. Add sulphur or lime to change the color.

*Party Animals—How do you prevent
and/or cure a hangover? Tell Dick.*

1. _____

2. _____

3. _____

4. _____

5. _____

6. _____

7. _____

8. _____

9. _____

10. _____

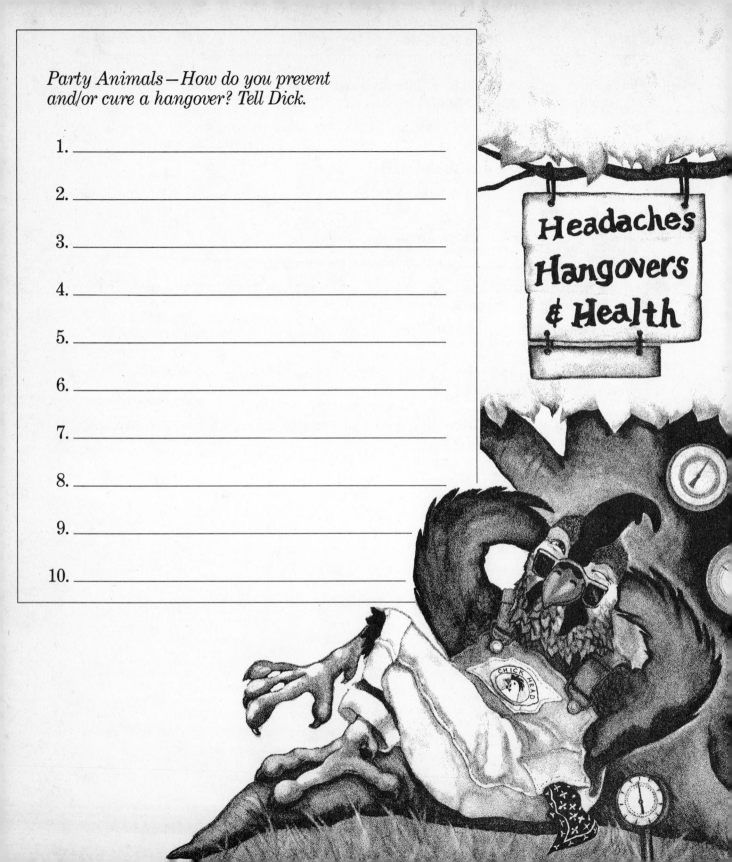

Headaches
Hangovers
& Health

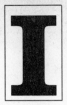

ICEBERGS — All icebergs are not white. Some are green, and some are black, their color depending on their age and place of origin.

ICE HOUSE — Did you ever wonder how many tons of ice that old ice house would hold? If so, calculate the number of cubic feet in the ice house, and divide by thirty-five.

ICE IDEA — Through the winter, set waxed milk cartons full of water out to freeze. As freezer-stored food is used up, fill the empty spaces with your "free" ice, thus helping your appliance to run more economically. In the summer, as you again stock the freezer with garden produce, the ice can be brought out for making hand-cranked ice cream, for keeping coolers cool, and for icing beverages.

IMPOTENCE AND SEXUAL PROBLEMS — In severe cases, a man should have nothing but liquids for twenty-four hours before making love.

Eat garlic; eat mint leaves and drink mint tea; eat celery, oysters, peaches, honey, parsley, and cayenne pepper; eat a cucumber a day.

Eat one-half cup of unprocessed (unsalted) shelled pumpkin seeds daily or, if you wish, try sunflower seeds.

Firmly squeeze the testicles daily, once for each year of your life. For example, a forty-year-old man should squeeze his testicles firmly forty times.

Drink four ounces of coconut milk every day.

Some people have good results by taking four bee pollen pills daily.

Take a cold shower every day for two months.

Take one-fourth of a teaspoon of ginseng twice a month.

To soothe the male organs generally, relax tension, and stimulate circulation, massage the area behind the leg in back of the ankle, about one and one-half inches higher than the shoe line of each foot.

In a circular motion, massage the inside of the wrists, above the palm of each hand, and/or the area above the heel and just below the inner ankle of each foot for two minutes.

Simmer one ounce of licorice root, two teaspoons of crushed fennel seeds, and two cups of water for twenty minutes. Strain and bottle. Take three tablespoons twice a day.

Reduce the amount of fats and cholesterol in your diet.

Quit smoking.

Exercise regularly.

Give up alcohol.

INDIGESTION — Drink some mint tea.

Chew a couple of sprigs of fresh parsley. Then drink a glass of water.

Eat one green pepper.

Eat a stick of celery.

Grate the outer skin off a whole grapefruit down to the white part. Spread the grated bits on a paper towel to dry. When they are crinkly dry, store them in a stoppered vial. When indigestion strikes, place a half teaspoon of the grated peel in mouth. Suck on it, then chew slowly. Soon your stomach will be back to normal.

Eat a large radish if it agrees with you.

Eat a banana.

Drink some white wine after your meal.

Scrub an orange and eat some of the peel ten minutes before a meal.

Sprinkle lemon juice on raw vegetables two hours before eating.

Chew some wild ginseng root.

Fix some peppermint or yarrow tea.

Do not drink any beverages during or after meals. Wait at least two hours after eating before drinking any liquids.

Make a paste of one tablespoon of arrowroot and enough water to make the paste smooth. Boil and then cool. Add one tablespoon of lime juice and eat.

To improve digestion, eat boiled zucchini with raw, grated almonds.

Bring one cup of water with one teaspoon of alfalfa seed to a boil. Let it steep for five minutes and drink one-half hour after a meal.

Add one-quarter teaspoon cayenne pepper to your food to improve digestion.

Add basil to your food.

To a gallon of water, add one cup of bran and one cup of oatmeal. Let stand twenty-four hours, then strain. Drink a cup of the liquid for fifteen minutes before each meal.

Drink a cup of water as warm as you can stand it the first thing in the morning and the last thing at night before going to bed. Always drink this on an empty stomach.

Drink a glass of hot water with a tablespoon of honey and two teaspoons of apple-cider vinegar.

Drink a cup of camomile tea.

Eat some papaya.

Do not eat for two to three hours before you go to bed.

Raising the head of your bed six inches should help if you suffer indigestion at night.

Lying down makes indigestion worse, so avoid lying down during the day.

Avoid these things that can cause indigestion: chocolate, tobacco, aspirin, coffee, tea, fried foods, onion, tomato products, garlic, citrus fruit, and spicy or fatty foods.

Eat slowly.

Do not wear clothing that is too tight.

Eat alfalfa sprouts, raw potato, or raw turnips to cure indigestion.

Avoid carbonated drinks, but drink a lot of water.

INFLAMMATION — To cure inflammation, get some strawberry leaves and lay the outside or the wooly side of the leaf on the affected area.

INK STAIN — To remove ink stains from carpet, take up as much as you can with a spoon. Pour some cold sweet milk on the spot. Then again use the spoon. If you have to, do the same thing over again. This should get the stain out.

INSECT BITES AND STINGS — Rub exposed parts of the body with fresh parsley.

Don't wear the color blue around mosquitoes. They're also attracted to wet clothes.

Rub exposed parts of the body with the juice of the aloe vera plant.

Apply the B-vitamin PABA and ethyl alcohol.

Apply a fresh burdock leaf that has been heated under hot tap water.

Apply vitamin C.

Dip a piece of cotton in cider vinegar, apply to the bite, and hold on with a bandage. In forty minutes, the itch and swelling are gone.

The juice of peach-tree leaves is good to apply to most stings.

Mix a little meat tenderizer in a few drops of water, soak it up with a cotton ball, and hold it on the sting so it can soak in.

Applying a paste of baking soda and vinegar or baking soda and witch hazel to the bite should reduce itching. Alcohol, benzocaine, or antihistamine drugs should also help the itching.

Caffeine also seems to counteract the effects of insect stings.

Pastes of salt, baking soda, aspirin, or tobacco or a raw onion applied to an insect sting should draw out the venom.

The scent of garlic, citronella, vitamin B_1, mint, orange, or oil of pennyroyal will repel insects.

You should wear drab clothing because bright colors will attract insects.

The scents of perfume and cologne will also attract insects.

Cider vinegar, safflower oil and cider vinegar, or a bit of butter or margarine and salt all seem to help insect stings.

Place a slice of raw potato or horseradish root on the sting.

Cover the sting with wet mud.

Mix equal parts of vinegar and lemon juice together and dab on the sting every five minutes until the pain is gone.

Apply a drop of honey from the hive of the bee that did the stinging.

To help control mosquitoes, plant castor beans.

Black pepper can also be used to get rid of ants.

Put a couple of bay leaves in flour, cereals, and beans to prevent them from getting wormy.

INSECT REPELLENTS – Hang a bouquet of dried tomato leaves in all the rooms in your home. You will not be troubled with flies, mosquitoes, or spiders.

Spray lemon juice to get rid of ants.

INSECTICIDE (CRITTER RIDDERS AND MORE) – Dry some horseweed leaves and use them in a smoker. Smoke your flowers and vegetables.

Strong sassafras tea sprinkled on flowers will make them healthier.

Human hair should be placed near trees and the garden to help control bugs, insects, deer, and rabbits.

Using your blender, add one quart of water and grind or chop three large onions, one whole clove of garlic, and two pods of hot pepper. Stir in one tablespoon of dish detergent after mixing the other ingredients. Strain and spray (except on edible foliage). If you have any leftover "mash," bury it between garden rows.

Mix one-half cup garlic powder, one-quarter cup of sulphur, twenty dried dandelion roots that have been cut into one-quarter-inch pieces, one-half cup of sugar, and one-half cup of borax with four gallons of warm water. Stir for three minutes, then let stand for fifteen minutes. Mash the pieces of dandelion roots. Stir again for three minutes. Drain off and spray this liquid during morning hours.

Mix one-half cup of garlic powder, one cup of unslacked lime, and two tablespoons of sulphur with four gallons of warm water. Stir for three minutes. Let stand overnight, then stir again for three minutes. Drain off the liquid and spray. (Spray during morning hours for the best results.)

Crumble some dried gourd leaves in one gallon of hot water. Add two tablespoons of cinnamon and two tablespoons of sorghum. Stir this mixture for three minutes. Drain off the liquid and spray.

Dried seaweed mixed with water makes a very good spray.

To keep deer out of your garden, take a shirt that has been soaked in perspiration and hang it on a pole in the center of the garden. Deer will not bother your plants. Of course, by the end of the garden season you may have a very ripe shirt.

Mix one-half cup of powdered garlic with one-quarter cup of Ivory liquid soap and four gallons of warm water. Spray on plants.

Take a handful of garlic and smash it into a bucket of water (a gallon or a little less). Put four tablespoons of sugar in this mixture and stir. The sugar is used so the garlic will stick to the plants. Be sure to mix well. Spray or brush on tomato plants.

A non-chemical way to control scale on plants is to use sour milk or buttermilk. Dab some on the infected areas and allow it to remain for two or three days. Then hose down with a sharp spray.

Mix one-half cup of garlic powder, one-half cup of sulphur, and one-quarter cup of Ivory liquid soap with four gallons of water. Spray on plants.

If gardens could talk, they would tell us what they want for breakfast: coffee grounds, eggshells, and fireplace ashes. Coffee grounds attract earthworms. Crushed eggshells are an ideal plant food, and fireplace ashes improve acid soil.

To make an oleander bug zapper, take a piece of lime about the size of a hen's egg and dissolve it in two quarts of water. Wash the stalk and branches of the tree with this water.

To drive striped bugs from melons, cucumbers, and squash vines, moisten ashes with kerosene and sprinkle them on vines.

Ant ridder: Mix equal parts of sugar and borax in a container, such as a cottage cheese carton. Punch a small hole in the lid (about the size of a lead pencil). Place the container where ants are seen. Keep out of the reach of pets and children.

Bug zapper: Mix one tablespoon of kerosene with one-half cup of milk. Dilute this mixture with two gallons of water. Apply the liquid with a syringe or spray. Afterwards rinse with clear water. This remedy is death to plant insects and should not injure the most delicate plants when used as directed.

Critter ridders for houseplants: Dip the inverted plant into hot water that will register 120 degrees Fahrenheit with a thermometer. Repeat on the second day. Do not allow the pot to touch the hot water.

I

Insect zapper: Hot alum water is the best insect destroyer known. Put alum into hot water and boil until the alum is dissolved. Then apply hot water with a brush to all cracks, closets, bedsteads, and other places where insects may be found. Ants, bedbugs, cockroaches, and other creeping things will be destroyed.

Mealy bug zapper: The mealy bug is also very destructive to hothouse plants. But they are really the easiest to exterminate. The mealy bug is a large, white, wooly-looking lump in the axil of the leaf and is easily kept down by frequent spraying with warm, greasy water to which sulphur has been added. But, if they are full grown, they should be picked off by hand or with a small, sharply pointed stick.

Protecting fruit trees: Garlic placed near fruit trees wards off certain insects and bugs.

Mulch your tomato vines and place them around your peach and plum trees. This should get rid of insects.

To prevent blight on pear trees, wind strawrope around the trunk to the first limb. Be sure this completely covers the tree to the first limb.

To keep deer from damaging fruit trees, buy some bars of Dial soap (it must be Dial). Cut the bars in half. Stick a wire through each half of the soap. Hang the soap from the branches of the trees you wish to protect.

For fruit-tree blight, mix one-half pound of tobacco dust, one-half pound of sulphur, and one-quarter peck of unslacked lime with four gallons of water. Mix well, then spray on trees.

Red spider zapper: The red spider is too small to be readily seen, but its presence is easily detected by gray or yellowish spots on the apparently dying leaves. The little insect lives on the underside of the leaf. It not only absorbs the leaves' vitality but also weaves a fine web that closes the pores through which the plants breathe. They delight in a hot, dry atmosphere, just such a one as our sitting rooms afford. But the spiders are readily destroyed by spraying the plant often with clear, warm water or by giving it a bath in the tub. Afterwards, sprinkle it with sulphur. If small plates of bright tin or glass with sulphur on them are placed under the plants in the full rays of the sun, no red spider will trouble the plants, as the sulphur fumes will kill them.

Ridding outbuildings of bugs: Buy some "burning" sulphur at the local farm-supply store. Crumble some paper into the bottom of an empty coffee can. Dump half a cup of sulphur on top of the paper. Place the can in an old skillet, placing the skillet on the floor of the bug-infested building. Make sure nothing burnable is nearby. Then light the paper. Close the door and other openings and stay away from the building for a day. The smoke fumes will drive out all the bugs and keep them out long after the odor has disappeared.

Ridding rose bushes of insects: Mix one pound of whale-oil soap with six gallons of warm water. Start spraying before bugs appear or as soon as leaves appear. Do this three times a week until the buds begin to open, then once every two weeks.

To treat rose-tree blight, mix equal parts of sulphur and tobacco dust. Dust on rose trees while dew is still on them.

Dust roses with white helebore while the dew is still on them.

Turnip slices placed around your rose beds will help in controlling insects.

Scales (*coccidia*) zapper: These critters infest cactus, oleanders, camellias, ficus, and tropical ferns. They are so small and so nearly the color of the plants on which they feed that they usually get a good start before being seen. Get a pan of warm water and a stiff toothbrush and go to work on them.

Root worm zapper: Frequently apply a weak solution of carbonic acid to the soil. Another good plan to kill these pests is to use water with lime dissolved in it for watering the plants. It also aids the soil in stimulating growth.

Slug zapper: Cut potatoes, turnips, or some other fleshy vegetables in halves and place them near plants. The slugs will gather upon the vegetables and are then easily destroyed.

Stopping cabbage worms: Sprinkle flour on cabbage plants while the dew is on them (early morning). As the sun dries the dew and flour, you will find that the cabbage worm is done for.

Treating blue mold on tobacco: Mix one-eighth pound of powdered ginseng with forty gallons of warm water. This should be enough to treat one acre. It is best to spray the ground before the tobacco is set. It is also best to dip the roots in this mixture before setting the plants. If the ground is not sprayed before setting or if the roots have not been dipped, then spray with this mixture after the plants have been set. This is a very good preventative. The mixture can be used at any time during the growing season.

Treating lethal yellowing in palm trees: Wild ginseng treatment is a folklore treatment for the prevention and cure of lethal yellowing in palm trees. The disease is spread from tree to tree and palm to palm by the quarter-inch leafhopper. This insect is green and feasts on the tree's circulatory system, spreading the disease. Follow these instructions:

a) Buy some wild ginseng root.

b) Drill a three-sixteenths-inch hole at a downward angle to the center of the tree.

c) Cut the ginseng root into one-eighth-inch pieces.

d) Place five of these pieces in the hole in the palm tree.

e) Use a piece of ten-gauge wire to force each of the one-eighth-inch pieces to the center of the palm tree.

f) Plug the hole and cover the plug with a mixture of lard and garlic.

g) Do this treatment once a week for six weeks.

Treating palm tree fungus: Mix equal parts of ginseng juice, walnut hull juice, and Epsom salt. Heat the mixture until it comes to a boil; let it cool until it is warm. Bore a quarter-inch hole in the palm tree at a downward angle. Fill the hole with this mixture once a week for six weeks. Be sure to plug the hole after each treatment. Mix a pinch of garlic powder with some lard and rub over the plug that covers the hole. This will keep out all bugs.

Wasp ridder: Buy three or four rolls of old-fashioned flypaper and pin them near the wasps' entrance. It won't take too many days for the sticky stuff on the flypaper to do its job.

I

INSOMNIA — Mix a teaspoon of honey with one cup of warm milk. Drink at bedtime.

Massage the spine with olive oil for thirty minutes just before getting into bed.

Read a chapter of the Bible just before going to bed.

If you smoke, quit. Smokers have a harder time falling asleep than non-smokers.

Place a wet towel to the back of the neck.

Drink a large cup of warm apple-cider thirty minutes before going to bed.

Mix one cup of honey with three teaspoons of apple-cider vinegar. Honey is a sedative and is digested by bees. Take two teaspoons of this mixture before bedtime. Honey will be in your bloodstream twenty minutes after you take it. If you wake up, take two more teaspoons.

Eat two small onions, raw. If this fails, eat a biscuit, a hard-boiled egg, a small amount of bread and cheese. Then drink a glass of water. You will now go to sleep.

Don't take afternoon naps.

Avoid coffee near bedtime. Caffeine reaches peak blood concentration within an hour of drinking, and it takes at least three hours for half the effect to go away.

Get more exercise.

Sleep in a quiet room.

Go to bed at the same time each night.

Honey combined with cider vinegar makes a tasty drink and works wonders when it comes to getting a good night's sleep.

Drink a small cup of warm ginseng tea.

Take a foot bath in very warm water and rub your feet well while they are in the water. Then drink a glass of cold water.

To induce sleep, mix together one ounce of peppermint leaves, one tablespoon of rosemary, and one teaspoon of sage. Store in a tightly closed jar until needed. Make a tea using one teaspoon of this mixture to a cup of boiling water. Let it steep for one minute, strain, sweeten with honey. Sip slowly. It would be better to use dried peppermint leaves.

To stop from grinding your teeth in your sleep, take calcium supplements.

Magnesium supplements seem to help people fall asleep.

Try relaxing before you go to bed. This can be done by reading, taking a warm bath, listening to calm music, etc.

Sleep with your head facing north.

Try using an extra pillow.

If you toss and turn, get up.

Go to bed when you are really sleepy.

Before you lie down in bed, breathe deeply ten times, count to fifty, then breathe deeply another ten times.

Peel and cut up a large onion. Pour three cups of boiling water over it and let it steep for twenty minutes. Strain the water, then drink as much of it as you can.

Place your feet in cold water for ten minutes. Then go to bed.

Press the center of the bottoms of your heels with your thumbs for three minutes.

Rub the soles of your feet and the nape of your neck with a peeled clove of garlic.

Avoid salt in your diet.

Eliminate all after-supper snacks.

Never eat later than 6:00 P.M.

Totally satisfying sex is a great sleep promoter.

INTESTINAL FEVER — Use a grape poultice.

INTESTINAL PROBLEMS — Try a high-fiber diet first.
Lay off the sugar.

IRON DEFICIENCY — A person with an iron deficiency will usually have unusually pale palms or eyelids.

IRONS (TO SMOOTH) — Rub with fine salt.

ITCH (BUG BITES) — Moisten the area and rub with salt.
Saturate a cloth in plain milk and apply. Keep the cloth wet with milk.

Apply vitamin-E oil.

Apply wheat-germ oil.

Lay off the sweets.

Apply sulphur and lard.

Treat the bites with jewelweed tea.

ITCH (JOCK) — Apply sulphur and lard.
Apply vitamin-E oil.

I

ITCH (RECTAL) — Avoid coffee and dairy products.

Apply wheat-germ oil to all affected areas.

Apply a wad of raw cotton saturated in ordinary vinegar at bedtime. Leave it on each night.

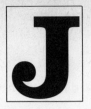

JAUNDICE — Try lotus-root tea.

JELLY MOLDS — Jelly molds should be greased with cold butter. When you wish to remove the jelly or pudding, plunge the mold into hot water, remove it quickly, and the contents will come out in perfect form.

JELLY TESTING — Add one teaspoon of alcohol to one teaspoon of fruit juice. If it forms a mass, it will make jelly.

JEWELRY (TO CLEAN) — Wash with warm water and fine soap. Mix one-half teaspoon ammonia with warm water and soap. Rinse with clear water and lay in cedar shavings to dry.

JEWELWEED — Crushed leaves and stems of jewelweed (also known as touch-me-not) applied soon after contact with poison ivy make a good remedy. It must be applied soon after contact.

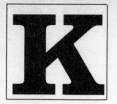

KEYS (PIANO) — Yellowed piano keys can be avoided by keeping the piano exposed to sunlight. (Ivory yellows in the dark.)

KIDNEY PROBLEMS — Drink a glassful of cranberry juice every day.

Drink corn-silk tea instead of water for six months.

Drink fifteen glasses of water each day.

Brew some kidney-bean-pod tea. Drink eight ounces every two hours.

If you have kidney stones, take one-half cup of cooked and blended or pureed asparagus before breakfast and before supper. You can also try eating nothing but strawberries for four days.

A medicine made from dandelion roots is good for kidney trouble.

Moreman tea (made of canutillo) is good for kidney and urinary trouble.

To help your kidneys work, steep watermelon seeds in a cup of water and sweeten. Take a quarter-teaspoon of the liquid every three hours.

Drinking horehound tea also helps keep the kidneys working.

KITCHEN HINTS — Zip up your gingerbread and molasses cookies by adding a bit of grated orange peel to the batter.

Light-colored molasses can be darkened to make dark gingerbread by adding a teaspoon of melted chocolate to each cup of molasses.

Don't risk soggy fruit or pumpkin pies. Just brush the sides and bottom crusts with the beaten white of an egg, then sprinkle lightly with flour and add the filling.

To peel onions quickly, plunge them briefly into boiling water and their skins will slip off easily.

Eliminate waste when measuring sweets by greasing the cup lightly.

Keep sweet potatoes from looking dried out by greasing the skins with any cooking fat or oil before baking them.

Apples stored with green tomatoes will hasten the ripening process of the tomatoes.

Mashed potatoes will look like whipped cream if hot milk is added to them before you start mashing.

Not all in one lump, please! Keep raisins, citrons, currants, or other fruits evenly distributed throughout your cakes by dusting them with flour before mixing them into your batter.

Save the water in which you cook rice. It's good to use in making gravy because it thickens itself.

Always sift flour before measuring it, and pile it lightly into the cup without jarring. Otherwise, you use too much flour, which is wasteful, and the finished product is not as good.

Save a piece of celery for the bread bag. It keeps bread fresh.

A teaspoon of salt added to the water in which eggs are boiled makes them easier to shell.

If baking meatloaf is placed on a slice of bacon, it won't stick to the pan.

Sticky dates, raisins, or figs will come apart easily if you place them in the oven for a few minutes. The wrapping paper can also be easily removed after this heat treatment.

Save the syrups from canned fruits for canned or hot puddings and desserts.

A full teacup equals a quarter-pint.

A standard teaspoon holds one-sixth of an ounce, and a standard tablespoon holds one-half of an ounce, three times as much.

Cracked eggs are suitable for baked goods.

To moisten stale rolls, place them in a strainer over cooking vegetables.

To make a crisp crust on homemade bread, place a pan of water in the oven as the bread bakes.

Homemade cookies will remain moist with a piece of bread in the cookie jar.

Waxed dental floss is a good twine for trussing your birds.

Herb aromas are strongest in the morning.

Pouring boiled water over your dried beans speeds up the soaking period to only a few hours.

Coat lemon juice over cut fruits to prevent browning.

One good way to save your vegetable water with all those nutrients is to freeze it in ice trays. Just pop the cubes into your soup as you cook.

Popcorn pops more easily when sprinkled with warm water.

Slightly frozen bananas rolled in honey and refrozen are tasty.

It takes ten eggs to make one pound.

Fresh green raspberry leaves frozen on baking sheets and stored in plastic bags make a fine caffeine-free tea.

A paper towel moistened with cider vinegar around your cheese will keep the mold away. Store the wrapped cheese in a plastic bag.

Keep your butter wrappers. They can be used to grease your pans.

Nonfat dried milk is a good substitute for nondairy creamer.

If gas in your beans is a problem, discard the soaking water and the first fifteen minutes of cooking water. Start over with fresh boiling water.

Another way to eliminate gas from dried beans is to add one tablespoon of castor oil per pound of beans or peas before cooking. The castor oil will not change the taste of the beans and will not act as a laxative.

A dried hot pepper in your jar of dried beans or cornmeal keeps out the weevils.

Add a drop of vanilla to a cup of coffee, and you'll never miss the sugar.

Put a pinch of salt in egg whites to beat them quickly. The salt cools and freshens the egg whites.

To make onions and potatoes easier to digest, put them in warm water for an hour before cooking.

To preserve meat, immerse it in molasses. It will keep for months.

KNEES (KNOCK) — Lie on your back in bed and cross your legs and knees tightly together. Hold them in this position for ten minutes. Do this three times a day.

KNIVES (CARE OF) — Clean knives thoroughly and dry them. Dust fine wood ashes fresh from the stove over the knives on both sides. Wrap each knife in a piece of cloth and roll it up in paper. Fold the paper over both ends. You may now put the knife away without its rusting.

Frymire's Kentucky Kontraption

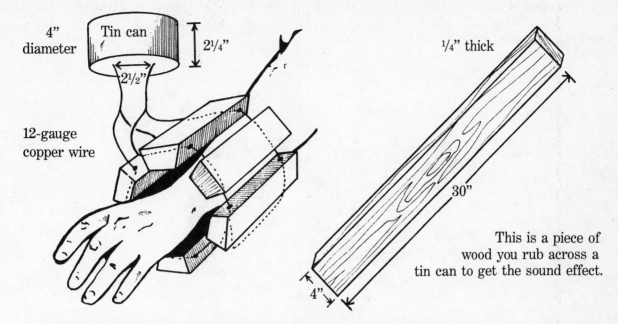

4" diameter

Tin can

2¼"

2½"

12-gauge copper wire

¼" thick

30"

4"

This is a piece of wood you rub across a tin can to get the sound effect.

This device helps to speed up the process of healing a sprained ankle, broken bone, or sprained knee. It also helps to cure headaches, etc.

Step One: Cut six pieces of wood ¾" x 1¾" x 8".

Step Two: Bore holes in each piece of wood. Each hole should be one and one-half inches from the end and big enough for 12-gauge copper wire to pass through.

Step Three: Cut off seven feet of copper wire for each side. Run this through the holes so that you have enough to twist together. Bolt this copper wire to a tin can.

Step Four: Each side will consist of three pieces of ¾" x 1¾" x 8" wood. Each side should be fastened to the tin can, which is to be four inches in diameter and two and one-quarter inches tall. The holes in the can should be spaced two and one-half inches apart.

Step Five: This can be used over and around a cast. Be sure to wrap or tie the device with string or strips of cloth. Do the same for a sprained ankle, knee, head, etc.

Step Six: Rub a ¼" x 4" x 30" piece of wood across the top of the tin can for approximately two minutes twice a day for ten days, then once a day thereafter.

How This Has Helped Me: In 1960, I had a knee operation that left me unable to run. The last part of December, 1981, I started treatment with this "kontraption." As of December 1, 1982, I have been able to run and go up and down steps without difficulty.

For Headache: Place the device on each side of the head and tie it securely. If, after the first treatment, the headache is not cured, wait two to five minutes and repeat. Your headache should be better or cured.

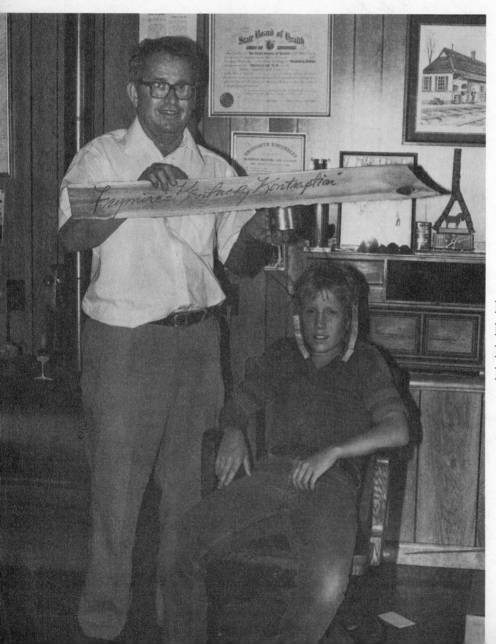

**Frymire's
Kentucky Kontraption**
Demonstrated by
Dick and Troy

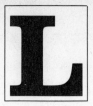

LADYBUGS — Ladybugs will kill brown mites and other pests.

LAMPS (TO PREVENT SMOKING) — Soak the wick in vinegar and dry. Replace the wick. There will be no smoke unless the wick is turned up very high.

LAWN MOWING — To decrease growth, mow your grass in the third and fourth quarters of the moon.

LEATHER (TO SOFTEN) — The best oil for making boot and harness leather soft and pliable is castor oil.

LEAVES — To preserve and use autumn leaves, carefully dry them flat. Take care to preserve their stalks. When they are thoroughly dry, varnish them, to produce a pretty gloss and to protect them from all insects and moths. Use the leaves as decorations. Store them in a container with a tight cover.

LEGS (CRAMPS) — Pinch your lip.

Massage your legs. Wrap them in warm towels or put your feet in cold water to help relieve the cramps.

Elevating the foot of your bed nine inches will help prevent cramps.

Drink two glasses of water.

When you take a bath, add a cup of ginger to the water.

To stimulate liver function, take coffee enemas and use castor-oil poultices.

Supplement vegetable broths with enzymes, vitamins, and glandular extracts.

Eat bananas and take potassium supplements.

LEGS (PAIN) — Try vitamin E and calcium to relieve leg pain.

To cure "restless legs," take folate or vitamin E.

LEGS (SHAVING) — Tuesday is the best day to shave your legs. After shaving, rub the legs with buttermilk and massage. Try this for two months, and you will find that hair will not grow back as fast.

L

LEMONS – Lemons, the citrus fruit with the most vitamin C, also contain calcium, potassium, and magnesium. They were once considered a medicine more than a food.

Mix the juice of two lemons in eight ounces of ice water without sugar. Drink this at 10:00 a.m. You will not crave food.

Lemon slices boiled with soiled white socks will turn them white again.

Cut a lemon in half. Then rub both halves over the tips of your fingers. You will then be able to remember things that you may have forgotten.

Keep lemons fresh longer in a tightly closed jar of water in the refrigerator.

If only a little lemon juice is needed, make a cut in the end of the lemon and squeeze out exactly the amount desired. The rest will keep better.

Keep pared fruit looking bright by pouring a little lemon juice over it.

Lemon juice, properly diluted, will not burn or draw the throat. This way it will do its best medical work.

Get more juice out of lemons by quickly heating them in hot water for several minutes before squeezing. You can also get more juice by rolling the lemon to soften it before squeezing it.

LEND – If you lend to the poor, you get your interest from God.

LICE – Wet the head with coal oil, then comb the lice out. Next massage the head with vinegar, wait five minutes, and give the head a good wash job.

Take one part lard and one part kerosene. Warm the lard enough so that the kerosene can be mixed with it. Stir the mixture till it cools sufficiently to prevent separation. Rub on the areas infested with the lice.

Massage the head with brewer's yeast, leave it on for thirty minutes, then comb with a very fine comb. Wash, rinse, and dry. Next slightly wet the head with apple-cider vinegar and let it dry. Wash again after two hours.

LICE (HENS) – Mix a handful of sulphur with their feed twice a week. The hens will like it, and there will be no more lice.

LINIMENT (FOR MAN OR BEAST) – Mix equal parts of laudanum, alcohol, and oil of wormwood. This is good for swelling and soreness.

LIPS – For cracked lips, use a very fine brush dipped in oxide of zinc to brush the cracks.

For chapped lips, dissolve a lump of beeswax in a small quantity of sweet oil over fire. Let it cool and rub it warm on the lips four times.

L

LIQUIDS – Sixteen tablespoons equals one-half pint.

Eight tablespoons equals one gill.

Two gills equals one-half pint.

Two pints equals one quart.

Four quarts equals one gallon.

A common-sized tumbler holds one pint.

A common-sized wine glass holds one gill.

Sixty drops equals one teaspoon.

180 drops equals one tablespoon.

LOCKJAW (TREATMENT FOR) – Do the following to the injured area: Put hot wood ashes into water as warm as the patient can stand. If the injured area cannot be placed in this mixture, wet some folded cloths (again, as hot as the patient can stand) in the water and ashes and apply them to the wound. Next bathe the backbone from the neck down with a mixture of cayenne pepper and vinegar. It, too, should be as hot as the patient can bear. This acts as a laxative stimulant.

LOCKS (HOW TO FIT KEYS TO) – Take a lighted match and smoke the new key in the flame. Be very careful and insert the key into the keyhole; press firmly against the sides of the lock. Withdraw it and the indentation in the smoked part of the key will show you where to file it.

LORE – If you chew dogwood, you will lose your lover.

If you smell a lily, you will get freckles.

LUNAR (MONTH) – A lunar month is twenty-nine days, twelve hours, forty-four minutes, and 2.8 seconds long.

LUNGS – As a remedy for lung ailments, bronchitis, etc., drink milk from a mare that is nursing a colt.

To protect your lungs from dust, get a piece of sponge large enough to cover the nose and mouth. Hollow out one side with scissors to fit the face. Attach a string on each side, wet the sponge, then tie it on. When the sponge is dry, wet it again. The dust will be very easy to wash out.

Rub some bamboo ash on the body as a treatment for lung conditions. Some even take the ash internally.

L

To check the condition of your lungs, draw in as much breath as you can. Then count as long as you can in a slow and audible voice without drawing in more breath. The number of seconds must be clearly noted. If eight to ten seconds is your total, you need advice. For any total less than six seconds, see your doctor.

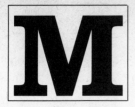

MALARIA — Plant sunflowers in your garden.

Eat cranberries.

Tobacco smoke is a fine preventative for malaria.

MAN — Every man starting in life should consider what his physical make, tastes, education, and habits of thinking and of life fit him for. Having decided whatever he is fit for, he should make that his life's work. No consideration of assumed respectability should cause him to turn from the bench or forge to sermons or briefs, unless his judgment convinces him that he has a natural aptitude or predilection for the new field.

MANGE — Use pokeberry roots and boil them down and give your animal a bath in the broth. One application should effect a cure.

MARBLE — Benzine and common clay will clean marble.

To keep marble from becoming stained, apply a hard, automobile-type paste wax to the marble surface and polish to a shine.

MAYPOP — Maypop (or passionflower, *Passiflora incarnata*) is a fine nerve medicine. Use a handful of crushed leaves in a teacup of boiling water and sweeten to your taste.

MEASURE (LAND) — One acre equals: 160 square rods; 4,840 square yards; 43,560 square feet.

One square rod equals thirty and a quarter square yards or 272¼ square feet.

One square yard equals nine square feet.

MEASURE (LIQUID) — Eighty drops of water equals one teaspoon, but different liquids have drops of varying sizes. A minim glass is a little glass tube or cup having a broad base and a lip for pouring. There are marks on the side and the figures 10, 20, 30, 40, 50, and 60 for so many drops — the figure 40 making one-half a standard teaspoon.

MEAT (ECONOMY IN) — Take leftover meat and cut it into pieces a quarter of an inch square, put the pieces in a frying pan, and cover them with water. Then put in a small piece of butter, pepper, and salt. When this comes to a boil, stir in a little flour and water, previously mixed. Have two or three slices of bread, toasted. Place them on a platter and pour the meat and gravy over them while they are hot.

M

To keep meat for a week or two during the summer, put it in sour milk or buttermilk and place it in a cool cellar. Rinse the meat well when you get ready to use it.

Meat can be made more tender by adding a little vinegar and boiling it.

MEDICAL HINTS — Sleep with your head toward the north.

Late hours and anxious pursuits exhaust vitality, producing disease and premature death. Therefore, the hours of labor and study should be short.

Take abundant exercise and recreation.

Be moderate in eating and drinking, following a plain, simple diet.

Keep the body warm; the temper, calm.

MEDICINE — To destroy the taste of medicine, take the medicine and keep it in the mouth. Then drink some water.

Always take your medicine while standing. Remain standing for two minutes. Drink a cup of water with each dose.

To make bitter medicine easier to take, suck on an ice cube for two minutes before taking it.

There is always a hazard of careless dosing of medicines made with herbs. Many are quite good, and there are many books that will help you in their preparation. People today lack the practical knowledge that old-timers had. They learned from experience just how much of a particular medicine to use.

Remember, most herbal medicines will need to be refrigerated when they aren't being used. If they aren't refrigerated, dangerous bacteria will invade the medicine. Even if a home remedy is harmless, the condition it's supposedly curing could be getting worse without proper diagnosis and treatment. There is nothing like experience and practical knowledge.

MEMORY (IMPROVING) — Drink half a cup of carrot juice together with a half cup of milk daily.

Eat four prunes a day.

Use fresh ginger in your cooking daily.

Pour one pint of boiling water over two tablespoons of dried rosemary. Let it soak for ten minutes, then drink the liquid part.

MEMORY (LOSS) — Cut a lemon in half and rub the tips of the fingers with it. Be sure that the juice covers the tips.

Bend over with your body erect. Try to have the head about belt high. Let your arms hang limp. Begin to swing them back and forth in front of you. Relax them as much as you can. Do the exercise for one minute four times a day.

MEN (HOW TO JUDGE) — Judge of men by what they do, not by what they say. Believe in looks rather than words. Observe their movements. Ascertain their motives and their ends. Notice what they say and do in their unguarded moments when they are under the influence of excitement. Know a man well before trusting him. Learn his habits and history; his reputation for honesty, industry, and punctuality; his prospects, resources, and supports; his intentions and motives; his friends and enemies; and his good and bad qualities. You can learn his good qualities from his friends and his bad ones from his enemies.

MENOPAUSE — Vitamin E seems to help relieve the problems of menopause.

Take three five-hundred-milligram bee pollen pills every day.

Mix one pint of Jamaican rum with one ounce of grated nutmeg. Take one teaspoon three times a day during your period.

Eat a cucumber a day.

MENSTRUAL PROBLEMS — **Excessive flow:** Steep a cinnamon stick in hot water and sip this cinnamon tea throughout the day.

Drink a cup of warm water with one-eighth of a teaspoon of cayenne pepper in it.

Steep two tablespoons of thyme in two cups of water for ten minutes. Strain and drink one cup. Add an ice cube to the other cup, soak a washcloth in it, and apply to the pelvic area.

Add the juice of one-half lemon to a cup of warm water. Drink an hour before breakfast and an hour before supper.

General problems: Calcium and magnesium supplements may reduce cramps. They should be taken each month before the period begins.
  B-complex vitamins should reduce menstrual problems.
  Calcium in various forms also seems to be good for treating problems once they occur.

To bring on menstruation: Eat fresh beets and drink beet juice.
  Soak your feet in hot water.
  Steep one tablespoon of basil in a cup of hot water. Strain and drink.
  Massage below the outer and inner ankle of each foot and the inner and outer wrist of each hand in a circular motion. Keep rubbing until the tenderness is gone.
  Steep two or three pieces of ginger in a cup of hot but not boiling water. Drink three or four cups of this tea a day.
  (Note: If you are pregnant, none of these remedies will work.)

MENTAL PROBLEMS — Sometimes the only problem is allergies. The person with problems should try wearing cotton instead of synthetic clothing. He or she should also eat natural foods, avoiding food coloring, additives, and other chemicals. A special diet without these substances could very well bring back that zing. See a medical doctor who is an allergist.

M

MICE — Plug up mice holes with soap. The mice will not go through.

Peanut butter works much better than cheese for luring mice to a trap. To make it harder for the pests to steal the bait, wrap about six inches of thread around and through a lump of creamy peanut butter before placing it in the mousetrap.

Bait your mousetraps with chocolate.

MILDEW — Mix two ounces of chloride of lime in one gallon of warm water and apply.

Fix a paste composed of soft soap, starch, salt, and the juice of one lemon and apply. Use half as much salt as starch.

Apply soft soap and chalk.

Wipe the inside of the refrigerator with a vinegar-soaked rag to retard the growth of mildew.

To get rid of mildew on the bathroom ceiling, scrub with a strong solution of chlorine bleach. You may need to add some trisodium phosphate in tough cases. When the ceiling is dry, paint it.

To remove mildew on fabric, mix together equal parts of denatured alcohol and water. Sponge the fabric and then allow it to dry, in fresh air if possible.

To prevent mildew from forming, place a piece of charcoal in a cup of water and leave it in a corner of the room.

MILK — Always sip milk in a leisurely manner.

Hot milk is a very good stimulant. Sip one-half cup for the best results.

Sour milk removes iron rust from white goods.

MILKWEED — Milkweed seeds yield finer oil than linseed. Its gum is as good as India rubber, and its floss resembles Irish poplin when spun.

MIRROR (STEAMING) — To prevent a bathroom mirror from steaming over, rub it with soap, then polish it.

Does your bathroom mirror get steamy when you shower? If so, hold your hair dryer to the mirror for a few seconds. In an instant, all the steam will be gone without smearing.

MISCELLANEOUS — The average body contains approximately fifty quarts of water and expels about four quarts each day.

If the cost of gas is a factor in your vacation budget, travel light. Every extra hundred pounds reduces gas mileage 2 percent. Those baggage racks on the roof increase wind resistance and raise gas consumption.

When you touch a flower, you are touching infinity.

A man in Iowa wrote me in 1984 and said, "If God created humans from the earth, the earth is the source of inspiration for nourishing and repairing the human body." He then added, "God doesn't make any mistakes."

If you touch your little finger and forefinger behind your two middle fingers, you can have any sweetheart you want.

Thomas Jefferson was the first president to wear long trousers.

Did you ever wonder why they moved the refrigerator motor from the top to the bottom of the appliance. The motors that were on top were almost 90 percent efficient while today's models are only about 60 percent efficient. Someone doesn't have a very good case of the smarts.

Since 1979, the United States has actually gotten more than a hundred times as much new energy from savings as from all net expansions of supply put together.

Laid end to end, the photocopies wasted each year in the U.S. would stretch to the moon and back forty-seven times.

There are 216 stitches on a baseball.

Be sure to appreciate whatever you are doing.

For each and every tree that you destroy, be sure to grow one in its place.

Attach a lightweight bicycle basket to an invalid's walker as a helpful aid for carrying necessities.

Sandals pinch? Dab the inside with rubbing alcohol and wear them immediately. The leather strap will ease a bit over the tight spot.

Couples whose forearms (measured from the elbow to the tip of the middle finger) are similar in length are more likely to have stable marriages. Short-armed women should not marry long-armed men.

Many people believe that the wood of cedar is sacred.

One key to our past and to human imagination lies in traditional customs and beliefs.

If the wind is in your face and the sun at your back when you are hunting, you will have an advantage over the game you are stalking.

Greed plus ignorance equals death.

Never spray firewood with an insecticide.

It is handy to keep a toilet-bowl brush under the front seat of your car. It is good for brushing out the dirt and dust and for retrieving small objects that find their way under the seat.

Cod-liver oil contains bromide and iodine.

If you get an insect in your ear, turn toward the sun. If you are indoors, turn toward bright artificial light immediately.

M

Ten inches of snow equals one inch of rain in water content.

All kinds of useful employment are equally honorable.

A neat trick for motorists is to save the last of the soda you stop for to clean bugs off the windshield. Carbonated beverages cut through grime and film better than conventional cleaners. Of course, you need to wipe the glass clean with a rag.

Serve that grouchy person some tea made from violet blossoms.

Take your handkerchief and soak it in water. Then hang it over a bush, rosebush, or flower to dry. When it dries, the initials of your true love will appear in the wrinkles.

Having trouble turning pages? Twist an elastic band over the tip of your index finger. Put another on your thumb, and you can leaf through a stack of paper quickly, turning one page at a time.

Be cautious of the ads that make outrageous claims for a beautiful body or easy-money schemes. Get the facts before you send cash. If it sounds too good to be true, it is.

The perils of being fashionable: Case #1—A young lady had suffered for months with tenderness of the tail bone, or coccyx. Physicals and x-rays revealed nothing wrong. Someone finally noticed that the young lady poured herself into jeans so tight that they embossed the flesh and suggested that she not wear the jeans for a while. It worked.

Case #2—A motorcyclist with the same problem was also cured by giving up his tight jeans.

Case #3—Tanning beds need special attention. They need to be cleaned thoroughly after each use. If they are not, you could be the one that gets impetigo, a crusty bacterial infection. Some say that cases of herpes on the buttocks have been contracted by using a tanning bed.

Case #4—Allergic reaction can be caused by wearing acrylic nails. This causes separation of the real fingernail from the nailbed, followed by an infection. A combination of allergic reaction and chemical irritation from the cement used to glue the false nails on is at fault. It will take at least six months to get over this condition.

Peel an apple without breaking the peel, and throw the peeling over your shoulder. When it lands, it will form the initial of your future mate.

It's no trick at all to button a stiff tab collar if you wet the tabs slightly.

Place a quarter-inch slice of onion in the palm of your hand. Then let someone place the palm of their hand on top of the onion slice in your hand. You could be able to tell something about the other person.

If you're a poor bridge player, everyone hates you and never asks you back. But if you're a poor poker player and lose a lot of money, then everyone loves you and you always get asked back.

Our country's young people aren't taking care of themselves. They have become highly passive, lazy, and wishy-washy. Most of them move like molasses in January.

MISTLETOE — Always gather mistletoe six days after the new moon.

Keep a fresh bunch of mistletoe in your home at all times. Place it where air from a heat register will circulate through it. Some people say breathing this air helps with high blood pressure, and it may induce menstruation. Some say it even helps in treating tumors.

MOLES (BODY) — Rub them with castor oil.

MOLES (UNDERGROUND) — Mix one tablespoon of castor-bean oil with two tablespoons of liquid detergent until it has the appearance of shaving cream. Add to warm water in a sprinkling can. Sprinkle the liquid wherever moles are causing trouble. It is best to do this after a rain shower.

Place Juicy Fruit chewing gum or cedar shavings and mothballs in the tunnels. Some people even drive small walnut tree twigs or limbs into the ground. One of these three things will surely get rid of moles.

A mole can dig a tunnel three hundred feet long in one night.

Broken glass will kill moles if you place it in their runs.

MONEY MAXIMS — When a mortgage on a farm is so heavy that the farmer never tries to lessen or lift it, the sooner he finds a smaller place the better.

MOOD RHYTHMS — Many people regularly go from happy to blue and back every three or four months.

MOON — The moon affects the minerals in the human body. This theory is based on my understanding that if the moon can turn the tides it can also affect the human body, which is 80 percent water.

The new moon rises at dawn; a second quarter moon, at noon. A full moon rises at dusk; a fourth quarter moon, at midnight.

A growing moon and a flowing tide are lucky times to marry.

Do you want thicker hair? If so, cut it during the full moon.

Never plant on the first day of the new moon or on a day when the moon changes quarters.

Do not schedule or attend a rock concert during a full or new moon. The power of the moon often touches the darker side of the human soul.

Do not have an operation during the time of the full moon. Bleeding is much worse during this time.

Castrate animals within one week before or after the new moon in any sign except Leo, Scorpio, or Sagittarius. Avoid the full moon.

M

MOON AND ZODIAC SIGNS — When the sign is in either the heart (signified by the lion on zodiac charts and on many calendars) or the loins (signified by the scorpion) and the moon is full or in the last quarter, conditions are especially favorable for killing bushes.

The day that dog days come in, all mockingbirds stop singing until dog days leave and will not sing very much for two weeks.

If the sign is in the head, wean the baby. He won't cry. If you catch the sign in the thigh, going down, he'll never ask for milk.

Do not ship a calf to market when the sign is in the head. If you do, the cow will bawl her head off. You have to get the sign away from the head and the heart before you ship calves.

Crops planted when the sign is in the bowels have a tendency to produce many blooms but little else.

Crops planted when the sign is in the loins don't want to grow.

The best time to plant, assuming the moon is right, is when the zodiac sign is in the arms, breast, kidneys, thighs, or knees.

Plant potatoes in the full moon. They'll stay beneath the ground and the vines will be short.

Potatoes planted in the new moon will produce vines two or three feet tall, and the potatoes will come to the top of the ground and sunburn. You can't keep the dirt on them.

Plant above-ground crops (grass and some corn crops excepted) during a new moon or during the first quarter phase of the new moon.

Plant underground crops during the full moon or the last quarter phase.

Gravel spread on a driveway during the full moon will sink. Gravel spread during a new moon will stay on top of the ground.

Don't run a line fence when there is a full moon. The posts will sink.

Pour concrete on top of the ground in a new moon, and it'll stay right on top. If it is poured on a full moon, it will sink and crack.

Cut burley tobacco in the new moon. It will cure brighter than if it were cut during the full moon.

Corn planted in the new moon is best suited for silage. It will grow tall, and the ears will stay close to the stalk. Corn planted in the full moon is more suited for grain because it does not grow as tall and the ear falls away from the stalk, thereby preventing water from seeping into the end of the shuck and molding the corn.

Ground is best plowed in the full moon. Grass and weeds turned under will rot and disappear. In the new moon, it takes a long time to decay.

MOONS (SIGNS) — **From new moon to first quarter:** Nights are darkest at the new moon. Germination and leaf and root growth are all stimulated. Plant quick-sprouting and extra-slow-sprouting seeds—those that germinate in less than a week and those that take about one month. The moon's pull increases to ninety degrees away from the sun.

From the first quarter to the full moon: Nights become much brighter as the moon approaches fullness. Leaf growth is stimulated. Root growth is suppressed. Gravitational pull is increasingly opposed to that of the sun. Do not transplant. Seeds that have failed to sprout in the past seven days are most likely to germinate during this period.

From the full moon to the last quarter: The moon rises later and later (waning moon). Nights darken. Gravitational pull narrows to ninety degrees away from the sun. Root growth is stimulated; leaf and stem growth, suppressed. Transplant larger plants and seedlings. Plant slow-sprouting seeds—those that take about two weeks to germinate.

From the last quarter to the new moon: Nights are increasingly dark as the moon rises shortly before the sun. The moon's gravitational pull narrows until it finally comes from the same direction. Leaf and root growth are both suppressed. This is a good time to ship dormant plants. Two days before the new moon, plant quick- and extra-slow-sprouting seeds so that they will germinate in time to benefit from the moon's initial waxing.

MORNING SICKNESS — Drink some warm apple cider. Take some deep breaths of air and exhale between sips.

Take fifty milligrams each of vitamin B_6 and vitamin B_1 daily. Eat garlic while taking these vitamins. (Note: Consult your doctor before taking these vitamins.)

MOSS (ON TREES) — To destroy moss on trees, paint them with whitewash made of quicklime and wood ashes.

MOTHS — A small piece of cloth moistened with turpentine and put in closets, chests, etc., is a preventative against moths.

If a few bitter apples are enclosed in muslin bags and put into drawers or closets, no moth will ever come near them.

MOTION SICKNESS — Suck a lemon.

Take the juice of one lemon, the white of one egg, beat, and eat.

Always eat a light meal before traveling.

Do not smoke, drink alcohol, or eat rich food before travel.

Powdered ginger may prevent motion sickness.

MOUTH — To treat a sore mouth, rinse out with goldenseal solution.

For an inflamed mouth, mix four tablespoons of apple-cider vinegar with four tablespoons of water. Rinse out the mouth with this mixture four times a day.

M

Eating a small amount of sauerkraut twice daily may also help an inflamed mouth. Be sure to chew the sauerkraut thoroughly before swallowing.

Eat celery daily if your mouth is inflamed.

Eat one-half cup of fresh strawberries three times a week. An inflamed mouth could improve within ten days.

MUFFINS — Muffins taste richer when the shortening is cut into the flour, as for biscuits.

MUMPS — Drink warm sassafras tea, and observe a very simple diet.

MUSH (FRIED CORNMEAL) — Bring to a boil two and three-quarters cups of water; combine one cup of cornmeal, one cup of cold water, a teaspoon of salt, and a teaspoon of sugar. Gradually add the mixture to boiling water, stirring constantly. Cook until thick, stirring frequently. Cover, and cook over low heat ten to fifteen minutes. Pour into a $7^{1}/_{2}$ x $3^{3}/_{4}$ x $2^{1}/_{4}$-inch loaf pan or any similar baking dish. Cool; chill several hours overnight. Turn out; cut into one-half inch slices. Roll slices in flour before frying. Fry slowly in hot fat. Turn once. When the mush is browned, serve with butter. Some people like syrup over it, too. Serves six.

MUSHROOMS — Take mushrooms out of their plastic container and refrigerate them in a brown paper bag. They'll keep fresh stored this way.

Mosquito Zapper

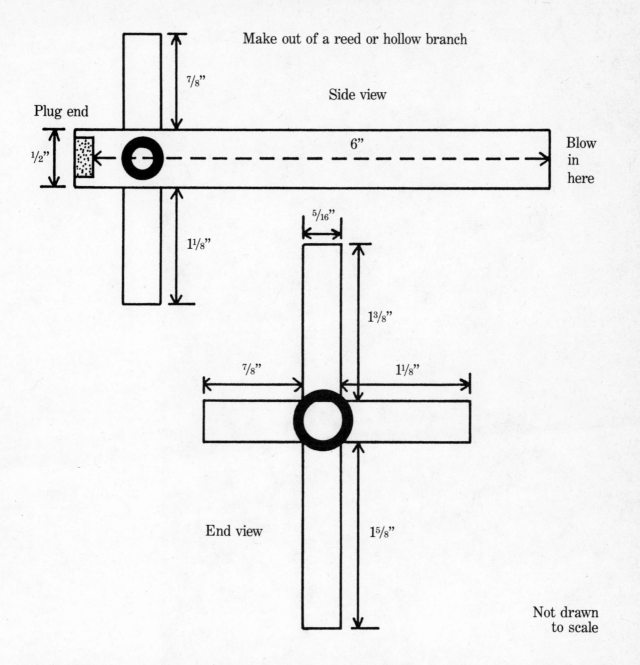

Make out of a reed or hollow branch

Side view

Plug end

7/8"

1/2"

6"

Blow in here

1 1/8"

5/16"

1 3/8"

7/8"

1 1/8"

End view

1 5/8"

Not drawn to scale

Hold a finger over all four holes and blow. While continuing to blow, slowly lift the fingers until you hear a hissing sound. Bye, bye, mosquito!

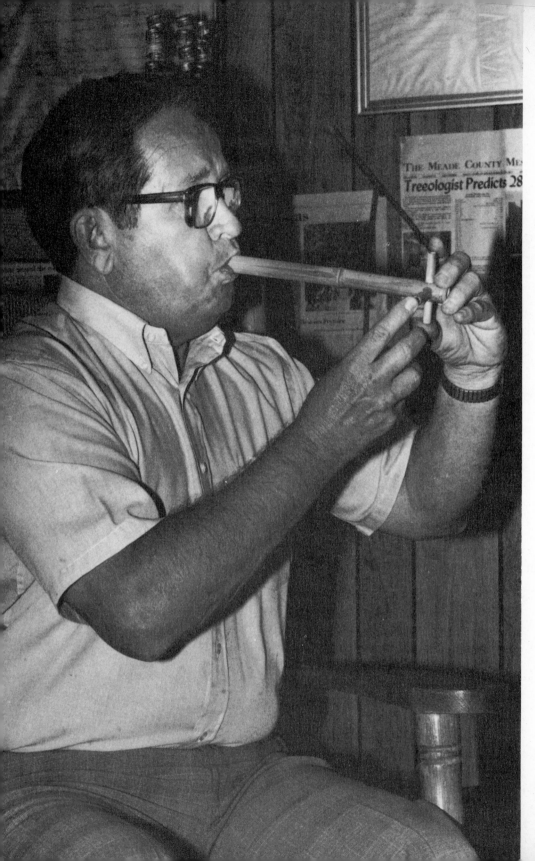

**Frymire's
Mosquito Zapper**

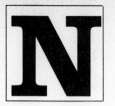

NAP — Always take an afternoon nap if you plan to be out late at night.

NATURE — All agricultural learning should begin with a study of nature.

Unless we heed the warnings of nature, in the not-too-distant future, the food-growing conditions of the world will change. Droughts and floods will occur throughout the world. The most fertile areas of the world will become barren. Just before that time, people will heed nothing but science and finances. None of us at this time can begin to understand just how appalling the misery will be.

NAUSEA — Beat one egg well (approximately two minutes) and add one pint of fresh milk, one pint of water, and enough sugar to make the mixture taste good. Boil and let cool. Drink when cold. If curds or whey shows, the mixture is useless.

Drink a cupful of warm water one-half hour before each meal.

Drink a cup of camomile tea.

Steep a couple of cloves, a cinnamon stick, or one teaspoon of ginger in a cup of hot water for five minutes and drink.

To treat nausea, gas pains, and dysentery, try one of the following:
   Fix a very weak tea from the leaves of the basil plant. Take one tablespoon every three hours.
   Take one teaspoon of pure cola syrup. Then take a drink of water.
   Crack an ice cube and suck on the little pieces.
   Cut an onion in half and place a piece under each arm pit.

NECK (ENLARGED) — To cure an enlarged neck, dissolve two tablespoons each of salt, borax, and alum in two tablespoons of water. Apply three times a day for three days.

NECK (STIFF) — Hot molasses and mustard make a good plaster for a stiff neck.

NERVE (PINCHED) — Bend over slightly, swing arms back and forth in front of you. Now circle arms to each side slowly. Do this for three minutes five times a day.

NERVOUSNESS — Your diet should consist of a lot of meat, and vegetables should be eaten sparingly.

You should go to bed and get up early.

N

Take cold showers.

Exercise will help to invigorate the nervous system.

NEURALGIA — Boil a potato in one quart of water. Treat the affected area with the water as hot as you can stand it. Save the water for further treatment. Crush the potato and apply it to the affected part as a poultice. This should be worn all night. In the morning reheat the water as hot as you can bear and again treat the area with it. This must be continued for several days, sometimes for as much as two or three weeks.

Heat a flat iron hot enough to vaporize vinegar. Cover it with some woolen material moistened with vinegar. Apply this to the painful spot. Repeat until the pain disappears.

Lightly apply oil of peppermint to the seat of the pain.

A quantity of bruised or grated horseradish applied to the wrist will sometimes relieve the pain.

Make a poultice of the leaves of common field thistle and apply to the affected area. Also make a tea by placing some leaves in a quart of water and boiling them down to a pint. Drink a small wine glass full of this tea before each meal.

For three nights wear a flannel cap that fastens under the chin. Skip three nights and then wear it again if needed.

Tie a strip of flannel around the head and rub equal parts of salt and alum on a soft, wet piece of linen over the teeth for neuralgia in the eyebrows.

NIPPLES (SORE) — Make an ointment of equal parts glycerine and tannin. Mutton tallow can also be used.

Soak nutgalls in boiling water. When the mixture is cold, strain and apply to the nipples.

Try applying a few drops of collodion to the nipples.

NOSE (SHINY) — Mix one-half teaspoon of USP fine-grind pumice, one-quarter teaspoon alum, and enough witch hazel to make a paste (about one-quarter teaspoon). All the ingredients can be found in a drug store. Spread the mixture on your nose. Leave it on for four minutes. Rinse with cool water.

NOSE BLEEDS — Try this very simple home remedy. Get a strip of bacon about three inches long, one-quarter inch at one end tapered to one-eighth inch at the other. Roll it in table salt, allowing as much to stick as possible. (It works better to dip the bacon in clear water before applying the salt.) Insert the small end into the nostril and push it all the way up past the affected area. Leave it in place until all bleeding stops (about ten to fifteen minutes). Remove the strip of bacon carefully. Don't breathe too fast for ten minutes. Repeat as needed.

Place an ice pack to the back of the sufferer's neck.

Immerse hands in warm water.

Put a piece of paper in the mouth and chew rapidly. Place a small roll of paper or cloth above the front teeth, under the upper lip, and press hard on the upper lip under the nose.

For frequent bleeding from the nose when there is no injury present, administer one teaspoon of vinegar in a glass of water three times a day to children. For adults, increase the vinegar to two teaspoons.

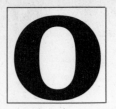

OBESITY — Mix four ounces of grape juice with four ounces of water. Drink thirty minutes before meals.

Eat Jerusalem artichokes.

Eat one-quarter cup of raisins and two figs daily.

Eat raw vegetables twice a day.

ODOR (BODY) — The following are good underarm deodorants:
    1) Dust with baking soda. Mix one part baking soda with two parts cornstarch for the best results.
    2) Apply white vinegar.

Take six chlorophyll tablets a day.

Eat lots of green leafy vegetables each day.

ODOR (CAR) — Place fragrant bars of soap under the seat and in the glove compartment.

You can place one of the fresheners made to snap under the rim of the toilet bowl under the dash of your car.

ODOR (COOKING) — Put some red pepper pods or pieces of charcoal into the kettle.

Boil three teaspoons of ground cloves in two cups of water for twenty minutes.

Heat vinegar in a pot for five minutes.

ODOR (FISH) — Fish odors from cooking utensils will vanish quickly if you add two or three tablespoons of ammonia to the dishwater.

When cooking fish, put about three pea-sized lumps of peanut butter into the skillet while the grease is getting hot. You won't have odor, and the fish will brown nicely.

Boil vinegar to combat fish odor in the kitchen.

Fry slices of potato in fat to remove the odors of fish, onion, or other highly flavored foods.

ODOR (FOOT) — If your feet smell, wear only cotton or wool socks. Throw away those synthetic socks.

Wear leather shoes.

ODOR (REFRIGERATOR) — Dip cotton balls in vanilla extract and then place them in the refrigerator in a small saucer.

Place one or two pieces of charcoal in the freezer.

Crumple pages of newspaper and put them in the freezer.

ODOR (SMOKE) — A dish of vinegar left standing in a room will dispel the odor of smoke. To get smoke out of the room quickly, soak a towel in water, wring it out, then swish it around the room.

ODOR (TURNIPS) — Lessen the odor of cooking turnips by adding a teaspoonful of sugar to the water. They'll be more flavorful, too.

OIL PAINTINGS — To clean oil paintings, wash them with soap and warm soft water. After drying them with a soft cloth, rub them with a silk handkerchief in front of a fire.

To restore the original hue of the blackened lights of old paintings, touch them with a solution of deutoxide of hydrogen diluted six or eight times in water. The spot must then be cleaned with a sponge and water.

OINTMENT — Melt unsalted butter and mix with a small amount of turpentine and linseed oil.

OLD WAY OF SAYING SOMETHING — Don't count your chickens before they hatch. New Way of Saying the Same Thing: Do not calculate on your juvenile poultry before the proper process of incubation has fully materialized.

OLIVES — Spark up the flavor of ripe olives by soaking them overnight in olive oil to which a very small clove of garlic has been added.

ONION (BAGS) — Onion bags, made of net, make great scouring pads. Crumple several pieces in a section of net and tie with string.

ONION (BREATH) — Leaves of parsley, eaten with a little vinegar, will destroy onion breath.

ONIONS — Onion smell on the hands or utensils should be scrubbed with salt.

Always eat onions if you are going to be exposed to extreme cold.

Hold onions under running cold water while you peel them, and there will be no tears in your eyes.

Always put onions and potatoes in warm water for an hour before cooking them.

ORANGES — To increase the amount of juice you get from oranges, keep them at room temperature or warm them before squeezing by holding them under the hot water faucet. This

O

does not injure the vitamin content yet gives you almost twice as much juice. Rolling an orange, lemon, or grapefruit a few times before squeezing it will also provide more juice.

A clever person saves some orange and lemon rinds, boils them in water for a short time, and uses the liquid in iced tea, lemonade, and fruit drinks. This costs nothing and helps make a fine thirst-quencher.

Before squeezing oranges and lemons, grate the rind and use it as flavoring for cakes, puddings, pies, etc.

ORNAMENTS — Suspend an acorn above a container of water within an inch of the surface. The acorn will soon burst open, and a beautiful ornament will be formed. The water should be changed once a month. Add charcoal to keep the water from souring, and if the leaves begin to turn yellow, add a small bit of nitrate of ammonia to the water. Chestnut trees can be grown in this same manner.

Take a half-dozen eggs, make a hole in one end, and empty out the contents. Fill the eggs with cornstarch made stiff. When they get cold, peel off the shells. Next pare lemon rind very thin and boil it until tender. Cut it in narrow strips like straw and roll it in powdered sugar. Fill a deep dish half full with cold custard and lay the cornstarch eggs in the center. Then put the lemon peels around the eggs to form a nest.

OSAGE ORANGE — This large greenish yellow fruit looks like an orange but should not be eaten. Some people call it a hedge apple, but osage orange is the correct name. The tree on which the fruit grows originated in Oklahoma, Arkansas, and Texas; it takes its name from the Osage Indians.

The trunk of the tree is short, and the tree features many crooked branches. The leaves are long and pointed and are a shiny dark green. The twigs are thorny, and the tree and fruit have a sap that is milky and bitter.

The fruit is good for ridding your home of crickets, spiders, roaches, and waterbugs. Place four Osage oranges at different locations in the basement. Put one in each closet and one under the kitchen sink. Keep the fruit out of the reach of small children. You will notice as time passes that the fruit will get smaller in size. After approximately three months of useful life, throw the fruit away.

OSTEOPOROSIS — We should all be concerned about osteoporosis—the thinning of the ernes that raises the risk of fractures in the hip, forearm, and spine. As we grow older, it becomes a very serious problem.

OYSTERS (IMITATION) — Grate six ears of sweet corn. Mix the corn with two beaten eggs and a little salt and pepper. Drop spoonfuls into a hot, buttered skillet and brown on both sides.

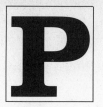

PAIN — Sometimes willow-bark tea will relieve pain.

To ward off pains, carry an Irish potato in the left hip pocket of your pants.

Mix some oil of wintergreen with alcohol and apply to the affected area.

If you have a severe pain in your hip, take a large potato and boil it in one quart of water. At night before going to bed, bathe and rub the painful area with the water in which the potato has been boiled as hot as it can be borne. (Save the water for further treatment.) Next, crush or mash the potato and put it on the sore spot as a poultice. Wear this all night. In the morning again boil the water that you saved and rub the sore spot with it. Continue the treatment for four days. You should be better by then.

PAINT — Rub your hands with mayonnaise before painting. This allows you to wipe paint off after painting. It will also leave your hands softer than commercial solvents.

Use shampoo or shaving cream to remove fresh paint from your face or hands.

To remove new paint odor, place a handful of hay on the floor. Sprinkle the hay with a little chloride of lime. After two hours, the smell will be gone.

Cut an onion in half and place it in a large pan of cold water. It will absorb the odor of fresh paint in a matter of hours.

Add a little vanilla to the paint to prevent that just-painted smell.

A neat way to keep paint from dripping down the outside of the can is to punch a few holes in the rim. When the brush is wiped against the edge, the paint flows back into the can. The lid covers the holes.

It's usually hard to tell whether newly mixed paint will match when dry. One quick, easy way to foretell the actual shade is to paint a sample brush-stroke on a piece of tin, then dry it quickly in the oven.

PAPERED WALLS (TO CLEAN) — Mix water and flour and make a lump of stiff dough. Rub the entire wall with gentle downward strokes. As the dough becomes dirty, cut the soiled parts off. Be sure to dust the wall before cleaning with dough.

PARCHMENT (TO TREAT PAPER) — Mix two parts of sulphuric acid with one part water. Dip paper in the mixture and withdraw quickly. Wash or rinse in clean water. Let dry.

PARSLEY — This herb, high in iron, vitamins A and C, manganese, and copper, is said to be good for the blood, the bladder, and the breath. Parsley should be eaten raw, or you can drink the juice.

P

PATENT LEATHER — Patent leathers are best cleaned with a dampened cloth and neutral soap. Vaseline will help prevent cracking.

PATINA (TO OBTAIN) — Rub buttermilk on a copper or bronze object to obtain this greenish effect that normally occurs only after years of exposure to the air.

PEARS — Poor pears should be given to the hogs.

PEAS — Don't add sugar to sweeten peas. It's much cheaper and tastier to cook peas with a few empty green pods.

PESTICIDE — Liquid seaweed is a good pesticide.

PHLEBITIS — Do not sit in one place for too long. If you must remain seated for a long period of time, alternating your weight should help.

Exercise regularly.

Taking vitamins E and C and lecithin should improve your circulation.

Vitamin E seems very effective in treating phlebitis.

PHOTOGRAPHS — Photographs can be cleaned by rubbing gently with a piece of not-too-soft stale bread.

PICK-ME-UP — Drink a large cup of cold or warm apple juice.

For that quick pick-me-up, try eating a few sunflower seeds.

PIE — It's as easy as pie to get a flaky upper crust. Just before putting the pie in the oven, brush the top crust lightly with cold water. The result will melt in your mouth.

To keep juice in the pie, mix the fruit juice filling with sugar and one and one-half to two and one-half tablespoons of quick-cooking tapioca.

A pie can be easily divided into five portions. Cut the big letter Y, then slice each of the large sections in half.

PIGEONS (HOMING) — Homing pigeons have three sets of eyelids, two of which are transparent, enabling them to fly through rain or snow and still have eyeball protection.

PILL (SWALLOWING) — If you have trouble swallowing aspirin or other pills, coat them with margarine or butter. With a gulp, they're gone.

PILLOW (DOWN) — A sure test for a down pillow is to hold the center in the palm of your hand. If the corners sag, get a new one because the down is worn and you're headed for nothing but insomnia.

PIMPLES — Eat brown rice daily.

Eat strawberries daily.

To cure pimples, dilute corrosive sublimate with oil of almonds. Apply to the face two times a day. You can also use a salve made from comfrey.

Wash your face with sugar and soap to clear up pimples.

PINEAPPLE — The top of a pineapple, planted in a pint jar of water, will sprout and root, soon making an exotic and most attractive palm-like plant.

PINWORMS — Eat grated raw cabbage three times in one day. Drink tea at the same time as you eat the raw cabbage. Do not eat other food at or during this time. Bye-bye, pinworms.

PLANTS — Every plant and weed is useful if we only knew how to use it.

Healthy plants on healthy soil resist pests naturally.

Plant magic in the Bible: An angel of the Lord appeared in the flame of the miraculous bush that burned but was not consumed.
 A balsam tree told David to begin the attack on the Philistines.
 Rachel was successful with Jacob after taking a dose of mandrake roots.

A good treatment for sick plants is to put several empty eggshells into a milk bottle filled with water and let this stand for several days. Then water the plants with this mixture.

Keep your potted plants in a very good health by using urea, which you can buy at the drug store, as a fertilizer. Use only one teaspoon to the gallon of water.

Here are a few simple tricks for keeping ferns looking garden-green and forest-fresh even in an apartment:
 1) Chop up two raw oysters and use them as fertilizer.
 2) Use cottonseed meal as fertilizer.
 3) Plant-food tablets, available at the seed or drug store, are also helpful.

To revive sick ferns, water with one-half teacup of salt to six pints of lukewarm water. If the ferns are infested with worms, stick matches into the soil, sulphur end down. For a plant of ordinary size, use four matches. Use six for a large plant. The sulphur does the trick.

To keep a house plant watered while you are away from home, cut a strip of soft white cloth an inch or so wide and two feet long. Put one end in a pail of water set slightly above the plant. Bury the other end in the soil around the roots of the plant. Your watering problem is solved for at least a week.

Chimney soot makes a fine fertilizer for gardens and potted plants.

Cold tea also makes a good fertilizer for house plants and acts as an insecticide as well.

P

To waterproof your flower pots, simply dip them into melted paraffin so that it sinks into the pores.

Garden tools will repay the care you give them. Protect your smaller tools from rusting by keeping a pail of sand near the garage or cellar door and plunging them into the sand when you are through with them.

You won't see insects on catnip plants. They secrete an oil that wards them off.

Loud rock music is detrimental to plant growth. Talk to your plants lovingly. Play classical music for them.

Plants are able to "sense" the sun without "seeing" it.

Plants can tell the difference between good guys and bad guys.

Try this: scream and yell at a plant off and on for three days. It will wither and die.

PLATE (CRACKED) — When you crack a favorite dish or plate, put it in a pan of milk and boil it for forty minutes. Not only will the crack usually disappear, the dish will actually become stronger.

POISON IVY — Apply vitamin-E oil twice a day.

Apply the fresh juice of the jewelweed (also called touch-me-not). The juice may also be boiled into a lotion.

Rub with raw rhubarb two or three times.

Rub with buttermilk.

Apply the juice from the aloe vera plant.

Take vitamin C.

Fels naphtha soap applied and allowed to dry on the skin seems to help.

Apply ammonia.

Apply apple-cider vinegar.

Apply baking soda.

Apply the inside of a banana peel.

Put orange peels in a bowl, pour any kind of whiskey on them, and let them soak for twenty-four hours. Take a hot shower or bath, dry off, then take the meat side of the peels and rub them all over the body, except the eyes.

Mix black gunpowder with cream. Apply to the affected area twice a day.

Mix some vinegar or buttermilk and salt and apply.

Apply willow-leaf tea to the affected area.

Run green tomato juice over the affected area. Or cut a green tomato in half and rub it on.

Slice a lemon in half and then rub it over the affected areas.

Boil four cloves of garlic in a cup of water. Apply with a clean cloth. Repeat often.

Take fatback and fry. Use the salty grease to rub on the affected area. If the grease is not salty enough, add salt.

Rub on bluing that was used to wash clothes.

Add some powdered white chalk to a pint of water and apply with a cloth.

Cover the affected areas with mud.

If you get poison ivy but you haven't been near the plant, it could be because your dog has brushed up against you after coming into contact with it.

POISONS (TO DRIVE OUT) — Drink May apple tea.

POKEWEED — Did you know the toxic substance in pokeweed, a plant that old-timers used for a number of ailments, has been shown to kill cancer cells in mice? Further research should be planned on its possible application to human cancers.

POPCORN — Popcorn is good for your teeth and bowels. It is not a junk food. It is the whole grain, containing the germ and bran. Popcorn isn't fattening unless you douse it with lots of salt and oil. A two-cup serving of fluffy kernels has no more calories than a thin slice of bread. Remember, if you want to put something on the popcorn, use old-fashioned butter.

POTATOES — Potatoes are healing according to English, Irish, and American folk medicine. They are high in protein and vitamins A and B, and they help neutralize acid wastes in the body. Because about one-third of the potato's nutrients are lost when it is cut before cooking, it should be cooked whole with the skin on.

Bake potatoes in half the usual time. Just let them stand in boiling water for ten minutes before popping them in a very hot oven.

Peel potatoes with a metal sponge like the one you use for scouring pots and pans. It's thriftier, easier, quicker. (The same idea works for turnips and carrots.) Rinse thoroughly.

Fried potatoes will be deliciously golden brown if they are sprinkled lightly with flour before frying.

POTATOES (A TREAT) — Cut cold boiled potatoes in small square pieces and dip them in beaten egg. Then put on a buttered pie plate in the oven and bake. When they are hot and brown, they are ready for the stomach.

P

POTATOES (SWEET) — A novelty hanging vine can be grown from a sweet potato by planting it in a hanging basket or pot of sand (or sandy loam), then watering it occasionally. The leaves are dark green and resemble ivy.

PREGNANCY — Take brewer's yeast to help with morning sickness.

PREMENSTRUAL TENSION — Sip camomile tea throughout the day.

Eat at least one serving of a food rich in calcium daily. This calcium should be obtained from beans and leafy greens.

Drink a cup of peppermint tea after each meal.

Add one teaspoon of garlic powder to a cup of warm water. Sweeten with honey and drink.

PRODUCTS (NATURAL) — Blossoms, roots, barks, leaves, and other parts of trees and herbs are as old as mankind. They were the main source of all drugs until synthetics came along during the present century.

At least 40 percent of all prescription drugs sold each year in the United States are made up, at least partly, of natural products. This percentage will be increased in the future due to rising fear that chemicals in synthetic drugs may have harmful side effects.

PROSTATE PROBLEMS — Eat one-half cup of unprocessed (unsalted) shelled pumpkin seeds daily. Sunflower seeds are second best. They both have high zinc content.

Drink five ounces of coconut milk each day.

Massage the inside of each wrist above the palm of each hand.

Massage the area above the heel and just below the inner ankle of each foot.

Drink corn-silk tea.

Take one pumpkin-seed oil capsule after each meal.

Take two hot sitz baths a day. Sit in six inches of water for fifteen minutes.

Some people have good results by taking four or five bee pollen pills daily.

Drink parsley tea made by steeping a handful of fresh parsley in a cup of hot water for ten minutes.

Cut coffee, tea, diet soda, tomato juice, and tomatoes out of your diet.

Drink apple and cranberry juice.

PSORIASIS — Mix one cup of sea salt with six quarts of water. Soak the psoriasis in the sea-salt water six times a day. Every evening pat garlic oil on the affected area.

Mix two parts of iodine with five parts of castor oil. Shake well and apply daily to the affected area.

Take lecithin capsules, nine each day, three after each meal.

Take vitamin E.

Apply vitamin-E oil.

Apply oil of avocado.

To prevent psoriasis, try a diet of fruit, vegetables, bread and other cereal products, and fish.

PUFF (POWDER) — Old powder puffs are handy for cleaning and polishing silverware. They won't scratch the delicate metal.

PULMONARY (COMPLAINTS) — When an effusion of blood from the lungs occurs, take a tumbler of a strong gin toddy.

PUMPKIN (SEEDS) — Plant pumpkin seeds with your corn. Set the seeds about four feet apart. This will discourage coons.

PUTTY (TO REMOVE FROM WINDOWS) — Melt some soap and apply to old putty. In a few hours, it will soften.

PYORRHEA — Mix five drops of iodine, one-half teaspoon of salt, and one-half teaspoon of soda. Brush and massage teeth and gums with this mixture twice daily. Rinse with clear water.

Eat lots of raw vegetables daily.

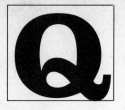

QUESTIONS — Do fertilizers alter the nutrient values of some foods?

Has the iron, zinc, and manganese content of grain dropped in the past few years?

Do you think that if the increased use of nitrogen fertilizers continues there could be a 25-percent depletion of ozone within a century?

Do you think it should have taken the government twenty years to ban DDT?

How do you know if something is safe to use?

Is the family farm on the way out?

Do you think life itself would be impossible without chemicals?

If a poison is lethal enough to kill insects in seconds, will it hurt a human being?

Do you think the answer to health will be found in the soil?

Is the condition of the soil in which our food is raised very important?

Has the use of pesticides since World War II decreased the pest population?

Are weeds and insects serving us in ways we don't fully understand?

Should crops be rotated?

Is the end result of chemical farming disease?

Do you consider diabetes a mineral-deficiency disease?

Dead Mule Valley — where is it?

Is sporting equipment becoming more important than the person using it?

Have you exercised your generosity lately?

Do people care for their automobiles better than they do for themselves?

Do we dig our graves with our teeth?

What excuse can there be to justify the fact that nutrition for animals is far superior to that for humans?

Should all high-school students be required to pass a test demonstrating that they have substantial knowledge about nutrition?

Do commercially grown chickens have arsenic and stilbestrol in their bodies?

Will the use of "natural" foods or "organic" foods lower the profit of the food industry?

QUINSY — To treat quinsy, an ulcerated sore throat, roast three or four large onions until they are soft. Peel them and beat them flat with a rolling pin. Tie them in a muslin bag that will reach from ear to ear and tie the bag around the throat. Have the bag as hot as you can bear it. Wear it at all times. The onions must be replaced as they lose their strength.

To relieve quinsy, boil a teacup of red sage leaves in a quart of water for ten minutes. Add four tablespoons of vinegar and sweeten with honey. Use as a gargle.

Spread tar on the throat. Cover it with a cloth and leave it on overnight. This should bring relief by morning. The tar stain can be washed off with Castile soap.

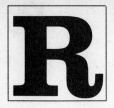

RABBIT TOBACCO — Rabbit tobacco (*Gnaphalium obtusifolium*) is good for people who have sinus trouble and asthma. Put the plants in the sink and run hot water over them. Inhale the fumes.

Break over rabbit tobacco growing in the wild. Point it toward your lover's house. If it dies, the lover doesn't love you. If it lives, the love is true.

RAISINS — Raisins for cakes and breads will be plump and juicy if soaked in warm water before you add them to the batter or dough.

RASHES — Use aloe.
For diaper rash: 1) Apply a heavy coat of liquid lecithin oil to the diaper area.
2) Apply vitamin-E oil.
3) Apply burned flour.
4) Apply honey.
For heat rash drink a lot of cold liquids and bathe in cool water. Avoid using creams or lotions that can block the skin's pores. Aloe vera juice, directly from the plant, is good for heat rash.

RATS (TO EXTERMINATE) — Mix two parts well-bruised common squills and three parts finely chopped bacon made into a stiff mass with as much meal as required. Then bake into small cakes. Put these down for rats to eat. Good-by, rats!

To run rats away, place a peppermint plant anywhere you don't want rats. If you do not have a peppermint plant, use a few drops of oil of peppermint.

To kill rats the easy way, cut a dry sponge into small pieces and soak it in lard or meat gravy. Place these pieces where rats can get to them. After they are eaten, the moisture in the rats' stomachs will cause the pieces to swell. Place a saucer of water near the sponges so that the rats can drink. Good-by, rats!

RECORDS (WARPING) — Place the warped record between two pieces of glass large enough to cover the full diameter and allow it to sit in the sun for three hours.

REMEDIES — One person wrote that she had suffered for four years from itching of the rectal area. She had been treated by several doctors, but nothing seemed to help. She told me about all the things she had used to correct this condition. I asked her about the color of toilet paper she used. My question seemed to upset her. I then told her that some people are allergic to colored tissue. She told me that she had been using colored toilet paper for several years. I advised her to use white tissue. She did, and within five days the itching stopped and has not returned.

Sometimes ammonia freely administered will help cure a snake bite.

If you have ingested gravel, eat fresh radishes and yellow turnips.

Eat onions and horseradish for dropsical swellings.

Tea made from butterfly weed (*Asclepias tuberosa*) is a good treatment for side pleurisy (a hurting in the side) or for getting over pneumonia or anything bothering your chest.

The osha plant is a good remedy for several ailments. Chew the dry root for toothache. Make a poultice for sores. Boil it into a tea for colds. Drink this tea for hangovers. Some say the plant will even keep snakes away.

RHEUMATISM REMEDY — Sunbathing can help.

Run through a food chopper—skin, seeds, and all—three grapefruit, three oranges, and three lemons. Add one quart of boiling water and let the mixture stand overnight. Strain and add three tablespoons of Epsom salt and three teaspoons of cream of tartar. Take one small shot glass or two tablespoons three times a day before each meal. This recipe will make about two quarts.

Mix together one ounce each of sulphur and saltpeter and one-quarter ounce each of gum guaiac, colchicum root, and nutmeg. This should all be pulverized and mixed with two ounces of molasses. Take one teaspoon of this every two hours until the bowels move freely. Then it can be taken three or four times a day until you are cured.

Take ten drops of oil of peppermint on sugar every four hours.

Cook cucumbers with a little salt over a slow fire for about an hour. Then press all the juice out of the cucumbers, bottle it, and cork. It should then be left in the cellar for a week. Apply to the affected parts with a flannel rag.

Bathe the affected parts in a mixture of one pint each of alcohol and water and a few red pepper pods left standing for twenty-four hours. When used, the liquid should be warmed.

Cut one ounce of Castile soap into small pieces, add a tablespoon of cayenne pepper to this, then pour one-half pint of boiling water on the pieces. Stir the mixture until it is dissolved and add a little cider brandy or alcohol. This should be used as needed.

Bathe the parts affected in half an ounce of pulverized saltpeter and one-half pint of sweet oil.

RIBBON (TO CLEAN) — Use one tablespoon of brandy, one of soft soap, and one of molasses. Mix together thoroughly. Place the ribbon on a smooth board and apply the mixture with a soft brush. Rinse the ribbon in cold water. Roll it up in a cloth until it is nearly dry. Iron. Do not have the iron too hot.

R

RICE — Rice grains will stay separate and white if cooked in water to which a teaspoon of lemon juice has been added for each quart of water.

Natural rice is one of the best foods in the world and is one of the richest sources of natural vitamin-B complex.

It is best not to eat white processed rice.

RING (COLLAR) — Do you have some shirts with a ring around the collar that you don't want to bleach? If so, just grind up some orange, lemon, and grapefruit rinds and rub the resulting pulp on the rings. This treatment will save money and get the stains out.

RINGWORM — Apply the brown juice from green walnuts every three days until the burning stops.

Wash the ringworm with lemon juice. Rub in a little gunpowder with your finger. Do this twice a day. Do not make the skin sore.

Mix five drops of iodine with one teaspoon of Vaseline and apply.

Apply full-strength Clorox to kill a ringworm.

Apply unheated castor-oil packs and rub with peanut oil.

Eat only raw cabbage and celery for two days.

ROACH RIDDER — Mix eight ounces of boric acid powder, one-half cup of flour, one-eighth cup of sugar, one-quarter cup of shortening (bacon grease will also do), and one small, finely chopped green onion to enough water to make a soft dough. Put small amounts into bottle caps or roll into balls the size of mothballs and put in places where roaches are usually found.

Replace every six days. Five weeks should do the trick. For heavily infested places, it may take nine weeks, but it will work.

Cut off some cucumber peelings and place them where the roaches are each night.

ROOFING MIX — Finely powdered charcoal mixed in boiling tar and constantly stirred till it is reduced to a state of mortar makes for a very fine roof. Spread to a thickness of about one-fifth inch.

ROPE (TO SOFTEN) — Boil in water for two hours; then dry in a warm room.

ROSES — Recut them each day. Use one quart of water, two tablespoons of fresh orange juice, and one tablespoon of household bleach or equal parts of water and either 7-Up or Sprite (non-diet). This keeps the water fresher between changes and also serves as a mild disinfectant. Interplant chives with roses to keep aphids at a distance.

Dick Frymire's Rain Machine

The idea for the rainmaking machine was given to me by an Oklahoma Indian tribe. A letter from the tribe described the machine used by their rainmaker.

First, they carve out three wooden logs about the size and shape of a fifty-five-gallon drum. They then tie the logs together with hide, taking a pole one and one-half arm's-lengths long (I figured this to be about five feet). Next the Indians roll out gold about the thickness of a number 10-gauge copper wire. They run the gold down each side of the pole, leaving enough on each end to connect the wooden bowl that is attached to each end of the pole.

Of course, I could not use gold, so I used copper wire. For the bowls, I used two tin cans. For the carved-out wooden logs, I used fifty-five-gallon oil drums.

To make the rain machine work, according to folklore, the rainmaker on the first day would place the pole in hewn-out log number one (the first barrel) and rub another piece of wood across the top bowl for thirty drum beats. (I figured this to be thirty seconds.)

The second day he placed the pole in logs number one and two and rubbed the pole thirty drum beats each. The third day, first, second, and third hewn logs; thirty drum beats each.

Legend has it that it should rain within twenty-four hours after the beginning of the first day. And if it has not rained within twenty-four hours after the last day, the rainmaker was disgraced and put out of the tribe, never to return.

The rain machine is one of my projects. Whether it works or not, I will leave to you to decide. Folklore says it does.

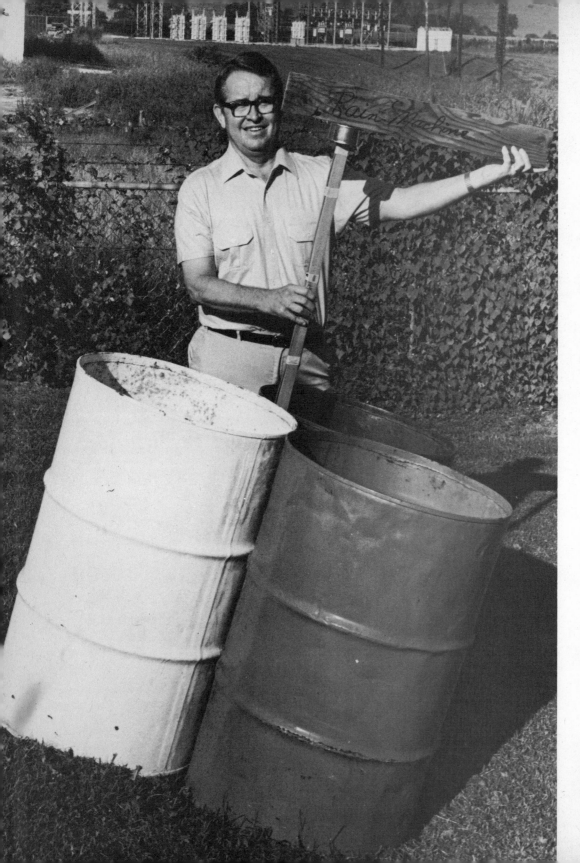

Frymire's Rain Machine

The Fry-Hut Relaxer

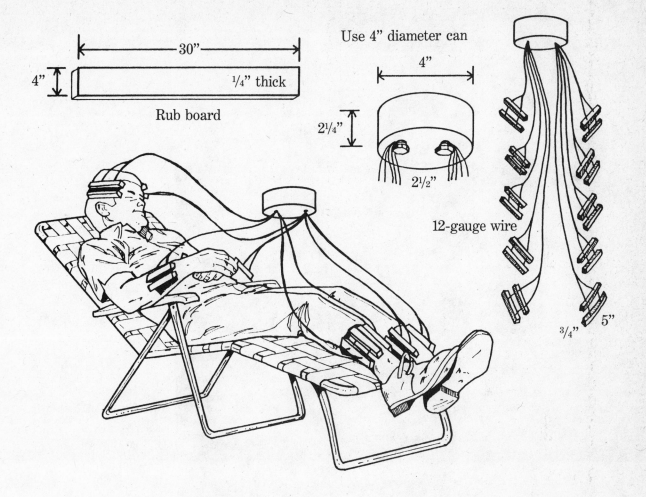

30"

4"   ¼" thick

Rub board

Use 4" diameter can

4"

2¼"

2½"

12-gauge wire

¾"   5"

1. Cut twenty pieces of wood ¾" x ¾" x 5".

2. In each piece of wood bore holes one inch from the end and big enough for 12-gauge wire to pass through.

3. Cut ten five-foot pieces of 12-gauge copper wire. Run these through the holes as shown in the diagram. Twist together. Bolt this copper wire to a four-inch diameter tin can.

4. Tie these pieces of wood as shown in the diagram securely to each ankle, each wrist, and each side of the head.

5. Rub a ¼" x 4" x 30" piece of wood edge-wise across the top of the tin can for approximately two minutes twice a day for ten days, then once a day thereafter.

This will help you relax!

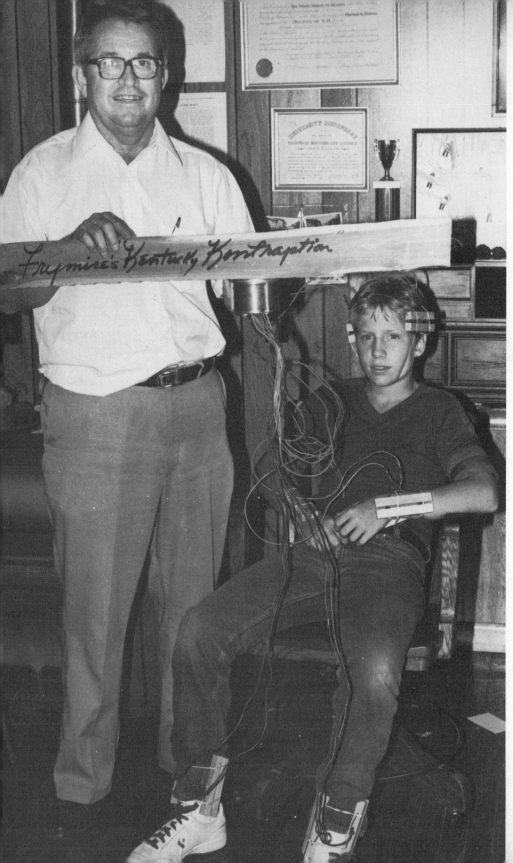

The Fry-Hut Relaxer

Dick and grandson,
Troy Jones

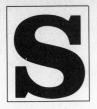

SALT — Carry a pinch of salt in your pocket for good luck.

Keep sinks, drains, and tubs free of grease and disagreeable odors by pouring ordinary hot saltwater through them once or twice a week.

De-salt that oversalted soup by merely slicing a raw potato into it and boiling for a short time. Then remove the potato, which will have absorbed most of the excess salt.

SALVE (BLACK) — Mix together one pint each of lard and sheep tallow, one-quarter pint of beeswax, one tablespoon of resin, one-quarter yard of linen (burnt black), one teaspoon of camphor, and just a little sweet oil or castor oil.

SALVE (WHITE) — Mix together one pint each of lard and tallow, one-quarter pint of beeswax, and one tablespoon each of resin, turpentine, and sweet oil or castor oil.

SASSAFRAS — Many people make sassafras tea in spring and drink it hot for a delicious drink. Many believe this is a good tonic that thins the blood and makes them feel much better. Water can be added to sassafras roots, and much delicious tea can be made time after time.

Sassafras bark, when boiled until a thick liquid remains and used as a shampoo, will kill head lice.

Strong sassafras tea sprinkled on flowers will make them healthier.

Chew a sassafras twig to calm you down.

Sassafras and dogwood twigs, when chewed, will whiten the teeth.

Sassafras poles make good chicken roosts.

Sassafras roots should be dug after the sap goes down. It is best to dig them about the first of the year. The best roots are red. Drink lots of sassafras tea in January and February. It will clean out your system and make you feel like a new person.

SAUERKRAUT — Sauerkraut is rich in vitamin B_6 and calcium. The lactic acid it contains will encourage the growth of friendly bacteria and destroy enemy bacteria in the digestive tract. Canned sauerkraut has been processed and has lost its valuable properties. If you cook sauerkraut, you should cook it over a low flame in order not to destroy these properties.

SCALP (DRY) — Massage the scalp once every ten days with hog lard. Allow it to soak for twenty minutes. Wash out with hot water and dandruff remover.

S

Apply warm olive oil and massage it into the scalp. Wrap the head with a towel and sit under a dryer for a few minutes.

SCARLET FEVER (TREATMENT) — Give warm lemonade with gum arabic dissolved in it. Lay a cloth wrung out in hot water on the stomach and remove it as soon as the cloth is cool.

SCARS — Rub with a camphor stick and then massage with olive oil twice daily.

Apply vitamin-E oil.

SCIATICA (LEG AND BACK PAIN) — Apply warm castor-oil packs to the lower back.

Eat fresh and raw vegetables, fruits, and fruit juices.

Avoid all meats, starches, and sugar.

Apply Epsom-salt packs to the lower back.

Drink potato or celery juice.

Apply a horseradish poultice to the painful area and leave it for an hour.

Take two garlic capsules and ten milligrams of vitamin B1 daily.

Drink elderberry juice and tea.

Massage the painful area with heated olive oil before bed.

Eat watercress, parsley, and alfalfa sprouts daily.

SCIATICA (SORE HIP) — Eat a handful of raw sauerkraut each day.

SCISSORS (TO SHARPEN) — Use them to cut a piece of sandpaper once or twice.

SCRATCHES (TO CURE) — A poultice of bread and milk should be applied for an hour or so and then salve until the scratches are healed.

SCREW (TO LOOSEN) — A screw that won't move might loosen if the head of the screwdriver is first heated.

SCROTUM AND TESTICLES — Apply a comfrey poultice to the scrotum to reduce soreness and swelling.

SEA SICKNESS (SURE PREVENTATIVE) — Make a mild decoction of bark of wild cherry about the strength of a breakfast tea and take a wine glass full before every meal for three days before going to sea. On the last day take a mild laxative.

SEA SICKNESS (TREATMENT) — Before going on board, take no food that is likely to turn to acid. Dry, hard biscuits with brandy and water are the best preparations for a sea voyage, and a little soda may be added to the water with advantage. Lie down as near as possible to the center of the vessel. Take a mixture of three tablespoons of camphor julep, thirty drops of ether, six drops of laudanum, and twenty grains of magnesia. The dose may be repeated after four hours. Keep feet and hands warm.

SEDATIVE (MILD) — Eat celery seed.

SEEDS — Rub seeds with sulphur and orange peelings before planting.

SELF-CONTROL — The value of self-control as a hygienic agent is very great. It prevents waste of vitality in feeling, emotion, and passion. It helps to give one a mastery over pain and distress rather than having those forces master us.

SEWER PIPES — Roots in sewer pipes can be eliminated by flushing rock salt in toilets and sinks.

SEWING HINTS — Store sewing machine bobbins in a clear prescription bottle with a snap-on lid. There will be no tangled thread, and colors will be easy to see.

Ease a sewing machine over heavy material by rubbing a cake of soap on the stitching lines. The soap helps the needle penetrate the fabric.

SHAMPOO (RUG) — Add one-half cup of powdered detergent to two cups of warm water. Mix until it looks like whipped cream.

SHEET-IRON STOVE (TO PRESERVE) — Rub once a week with a piece of flannel wet with a few drops of oil or melted lard.

SHINGLES — Mix two drops of iodine and one teaspoon of apple-cider vinegar and two pinches of sulphur. Apply as needed. Some people will increase the amount of iodine, using three, four, or five drops instead of two.

Take four vitamin-E capsules (four hundreds units each) daily and rub vitamin-E oil on the blisters. This has helped in many cases.

Apply the juice of the aloe vera plant.

Apply a paste of Epsom salt and water.

Drink one and one-half quarts of celery juice daily.

Mix two tablespoons of vinegar with one-half cup of buttermilk. Rub this mixture on the sore place twice a day for ten days, then once a day thereafter.

Eat a high-fiber diet.

Mix one tablespoon of vinegar and one tablespoon of honey with eight ounces of water and drink with each meal.

Mix five drops of iodine with one tablespoon of castor oil and apply.

Drink watermelon-seed tea.

Place an ice pack over the affected area.

Place warm soda water packs over the affected area.

Eat fruits and raw and cooked vegetables and drink their juices.

Avoid sweets, alcohol, meats, and apples.

Avoid citrus-cereal combinations.

SHOES — Polish scuffed shoes with banana peelings.

To prevent new shoes from slipping, sandpaper the soles.

Silence squeaking shoes by piercing the sole with three or four little holes, right behind the ball of the foot.

Rub a few drops of lemon juice into the leather to shine shoes.

SIGNS — In a barber shop: Clip Joint.

In a bar: Remember, the customer is always tight.

In a garage: Wanted, man to work eight hours to replace the man who didn't.

In a factory: Look alive, you can be replaced by a button.

On a Kentucky restaurant: House of grill repute.

In a maternity ward: Call us any time of the night or day. We deliver.

In a Georgia nursery: Plant parenthood.

In a school hallway: Free Monday through Friday: Knowledge. Bring your own container.

On the door of a music store: Gone Chopin. Be Bach soon. Offenbach in a few minutes.

SILVERWARE — Use the water in which potatoes have been boiled to wash silverware.

Never allow a particle of soap to touch silverware.

Soak tarnished silverware in a mixture of one teaspoon of soda and one teaspoon of salt per quart of water in an enameled dishpan.

Polish silver knives with charcoal powder.

SINUS (TROUBLE) — Gently inhale the vapors of freshly grated horseradish.

Mix equal amounts of lemon juice and grated horseradish. Eat one teaspoon one hour before breakfast and one hour after supper.

To stop sniffles, swallow one teaspoon of honey with freshly ground pepper sprinkled on it. Do not inhale the pepper as you take the honey.

Take three garlic perles in the morning and three in the evening.

Drop a couple of drops of vitamin E in each nostril, night and morning. After each treatment, lie down with your head back for five minutes.

To zap sinus infection pain, use a weak table salt solution in an eye cup and suction up through each nostril, through the sinus, and into the mouth. After each sinus is washed out, use a forty-watt light bulb on a small cord with a light switch to turn the light off and on to control heat. Wrap the light bulb in a thin undershirt and apply heat to all areas around the eyes and nose. Do this every four hours for as many days as needed. This cleans, heals, and gives complete relief.

SKIN PROBLEMS – Wash with cool or warm water; do not use hot water.

Take your bath or shower at night before bed rather than in the morning.

Grow plants that require a lot of water, such as ferns and large-leaved plants, which give off moisture.

Use food shortening to keep your skin soft and smooth.

To toughen sensitive skin, soak in a very strong tea.

Apply olive, safflower, cod-liver, and mineral oils for dry skin.

For cleaner skin, mix cornmeal and hand-rolled oatmeal with milk or cream to make a paste and rub it on your skin. Wash this off with warm water after thirty minutes.

To make a mask that will tighten the skin, whip two egg whites until they are frothy and spread them on your clean face. Avoid the area under the eyes.

Aging Skin: Rub with cucumber juice and olive oil.
Drink sassafras tea.
Massage the skin with pure creamy butter. This is especially good for dry skin.

Itching Skin: Mix one or two cups of baking soda with a tub full of water. Get in and soak for twenty or thirty minutes. While in the water, keep stirring the soda.
After you have drawn your bath water, add two tablespoons of olive oil. Take your bath and pat dry when you are finished.
If you take showers, before you dry off, apply a small amount of olive oil (one-half teaspoon) to your body.

Spots on Skin: Mix some flour of sulphur in a little milk and let it stand for three hours. After three hours without disturbing the sulphur, use the milk as a lotion. Rub this lotion into the skin with a cloth. Wash the skin with soap and water. Cold cream should be rubbed in at bedtime. It won't take long for the spots to disappear.

Rub brown skin spots with castor oil and watch them fade away.

SLUGS — Place garlic in any place where you don't want slugs. They won't come near the smell.

Spray the area where slugs are a problem with fresh lime juice. Strain it before putting it in the sprayer to prevent the nozzle from clogging.

To catch slugs, put a dish of beer in the garden at night. They will desert the plants and drown in the brew.

SMOKING — If you want to stop smoking or to cut down, suck on a small clove. You may need to replace the clove every two hours.

SNACKS — If you must snack, try these: carrots, a piece of raw potato or cabbage, a small handful of raisins, peanuts in the shell, popcorn with no salt or butter, apples, celery. Raw onions are also a very fine snack. Remember to eat or chew a small piece of sassafras root bark or parsley after eating onions. These two things will kill onion breath.

SNAILS — Snails and slugs won't cross a line of lime.

SNAKES (UNDER HOUSE) — Purchase an ounce of peppermint oil at your local drug store. Take a medicine dropper and place one drop every two feet till you circle the house.

SNEEZING — Put your finger on the tip of your nose and press in.

Breathe some rubbing alcohol fumes.

SNOWDRIFT REMEDY — Keep four three-foot long shingles in your car year round, just so you'll never be caught in a snowdrift or an icy spot without a means of traction. It's easy to slide two tire-width shingles—abrasive side up—under each of the drive wheels for six feet of no-skid pull. The shingles can be stored in a small space and are light enough for anyone to use. No instructions are needed.

SOAKING (CLOTHING) — If you must soak clothing before washing, limit it to fifteen minutes in cool water with light suds.

SOAP MAKING — Soap will be firm and white when it's made in the light of the moon. A sassafras limb must be used to stir the soap while it is making.

SOCK — You can judge a child's sock size by wrapping the foot of the sock around the child's fist. If the toe and heel meet easily, the size is right.

SODA (BAKING) — The dictionary defines it as a "water soluble powder $NaHCO_3$." I call it a safe and useful miracle worker.

Soda makes an excellent powder for brushing your teeth.

Offer your family hot-from-the-stove soda biscuits. They are delicious and inexpensive.

Baking soda is excellent for removing stains from coffee cups and glass percolators. It is also good for cleaning countertops and bath tubs, including fiberglass, without scratching.

A good, all-purpose cleanser can be made by mixing one-half cup of ammonia, one-half cup of white vinegar, and one-quarter cup of baking soda in one-half gallon of water. Wet a stiff nailbrush with the solution. This is good for removing spots from carpet. A sponge saturated with the liquid removes smudges from walls and woodwork.

Wash down shower walls with the solution.

To clean drains, pour one-half cup of soda followed by one-half cup of vinegar (add a dash of salt to cut the grease) down the drain. Wait one-half hour and flush well with water. Do this weekly. If you have a septic tank, a cup of soda once a week will neutralize pH and encourage helpful bacteria.

Add a little less detergent and make up the difference with dry baking soda to produce a cleaner, softer laundry.

To remove acid from car battery terminals, make a paste of soda and water and apply it to the terminals. Let it stand for a few minutes and wipe off.

If your face is reddened by the sun, wash it with a soothing solution of baking soda.

Dab bee stings with a soda-and-water paste to relieve pain.

If your grapes are ripening, put four teaspoons of soda in a gallon of water. Spray the fruit once a week to alkalize skins and keep down fungus.

Add one-half cup of soda to your bath water for a soft, refreshing bath.

Extinguish grease fires on your stove by tossing a handful of soda on the flames. When heated, soda releases carbon dioxide and prevents further combustion. Never throw water on a kitchen stove fire!

While washing dishes, if you find something burnt on the bottom of a pan, cover it with baking soda paste. Let it stand overnight. It will be easy to wash off the next morning.

If you feel queasy after eating greasy food, put one-half teaspoon of bicarbonate in water and drink. People with high blood pressure should not make this a habit because of soda's high sodium content.

Refrigerators can be cleaned with a weak solution of baking soda.

Always put a pinch of soda in sea water before washing clothes in it.

S

A pinch of baking soda added to powdered sugar icing keeps it moist.

SODA (LOW-CALORIE) — Make your own low-calorie soda by filling a glass three-quarters full of club soda and adding unsweetened fruit juice.

SODIUM (LOWERING INTAKE) — One easy way to lower your sodium intake and also keep your food flavorful is to switch the tops of the shakers! Less salt, more pepper.

SOIL (TO TEST) — To test your soil, plant garlic. If the garlic grows well, your soil is rich.

SOME THINGS TO KNOW — A small boy is an accessory to the grime.

A carpenter does his level best.

Old policemen never die. They just cop out.

Old gardeners never die. They just spade away.

Old teachers never die. They just lose their class.

Old checker players never die. They just move away.

Your brain is no stronger than its weakest think.

Old burglars never die. They just steal away into the night.

A kindergarten teacher is a woman who knows how to make little things count.

Frown. At least you'll get credit for thinking.

Success is merely a matter of putting your knows to the grindstone.

A bachelor is a fellow who failed to embrace his opportunities.

In the old days, a naughty child was straightened up by being bent over.

Prejudice is being positive about something negative.

You shouldn't judge a modern girl by her clothes. There really isn't enough evidence.

Etiquette is learning to yawn with your mouth closed.

Words are losing all their meaning . . . like zip in zip code.

A diplomat is anyone who thinks twice before saying nothing.

SORES AND BURNS — Mix powdered alum with Vaseline and apply.

SORE SPOT — Place a flat-iron on the stove until the iron is hot. Moisten some woolen fabric or cloth with vinegar. Cover the flat-iron with this moistened cloth. Apply at once to the sore spot. Do this four times in one day. The second day the pain will be gone.

SORE THROAT — Place a cloth wrung out from cold water around the neck at night.

Hold some powdered alum in your mouth and let it melt, then slowly swallow it.

Gargle with salt and vinegar to which a little cayenne pepper has been added.

Strong whiskey rubbed upon the throat (outside) often relieves sore throat. After rubbing the throat, cover it quickly with a cloth.

Simmer red pepper, honey or sugar, and vinegar together, tempered with a little water. This is a good remedy for a sore throat.

SOUPS — A little oatmeal adds much flavor and richness when used as a thickener for soups. Try it.

SPOTS AND STAINS (TO REMOVE) —Acid: Wash and rinse several times in cold water. Apply a few drops of ammonia and sponge with water. Launder in the regular way. If the acid has affected the color of the garment, white vinegar can sometimes restore it.

Adhesive tape marks: As a rule, they come off easily with a few dabs of non-flammable dry-cleaning fluid.

Alcohol and paint stains: Sponge with turpentine and then launder.

Automobile grease: Scrape off excess. If the garment is washable, rub lard into the spot until no more grease is picked up. Then scrape off the lard and launder. If the garment is not washable, sponge with non-flammable dry-cleaning fluid.

Blood stains: If the stain is fresh, soak the garment in cold water. Wash in warm suds. For a stubborn stain, use a saltwater solution (one-quarter cup of salt to two cups of water). Do not use hot water first. It will set the stain.

Butter: Launder in warm, soapy water.

Candy stains (other than chocolate): Soak in hot water or rub with a clean cloth dampened with very hot water.

Chewing gum: Rub with a piece of ice and scrape off the gum. If the stain remains, sponge with carbon tetrachloride or another solvent.

Cleaning fluid: Steam the fabric over a teakettle.

Coffee: Pour boiling water from a height of two feet through the stain. If this doesn't work, bleach with hydrogen peroxide. Rinse well. Do not use soap first. It may set the stain. For old coffee stains, use chlorine bleach, unless the color of the fabric is affected by the bleach. Test a small swatch from an inconspicuous part of the garment first.

Cream: Soak in cold water. Wash in warm suds. Rinse well.

Egg stains: Do not use hot water. Soak fabrics in cold water, then wash. On fixed surfaces, let the egg dry and scrape off with a blunt knife. Sponge with carbon tetrachloride if greasy, then sponge with cold water.

Fingermarks (on felt hats): Rub very fine sandpaper gently with the nap of the felt until the fingermarks disappear.

Fruit or fruit juices: Pour boiling water from a height of two feet through the stain. If the stain is not removed, use hydrogen peroxide. Rinse well. Do not use soap first. It may set the stain. Hot sweet milk will remove fruit stains when used before soap is applied.

Glue: Soak in warm water and boil if necessary. For non-washable materials, sponging with non-flammable cleaning fluid is effective.

Grass: Rub with grease (cooking oil) and wash in hot suds. Bleach any remaining stain with hydrogen peroxide. Rinse well.

Gravy: Iron out grease between blotters.

Grease: Rub well with soap and soiled spots with French chalk. Let stand for a few hours. Then brush off. Repeat the application if necessary.

To remove a grease stain from polyester, rub with talcum powder. Let it stand for twelve hours, then brush off.

Ice cream: Soak in cold water. If the ice cream is fruit, berry, or chocolate, treat the stain as such. Wash in warm suds. Rinse well.

Ink: Soak in cold water. Then apply vinegar or lemon juice. Bleach remaining stains with oxalic-acid solution. Rinse well. Alternate this solution with diluted ammonia. Or soak in sour milk and wash in hot suds.

Iron rust: Soak in oxalic-acid solution. When the stain disappears, apply a weak ammonia solution. Rinse well. Or moisten with lemon juice and salt and dry in the sun.

Lipstick or rouge: Rub with lard or Vaseline. Wash in hot suds. If the stain remains, bleach with hydrogen peroxide. Do not use soap first. It may set the stain.

Mercurochrome: Flush out with clear water. Treat the remaining stain with chlorine bleach if the color of the fabric is not affected by bleach.

Nail polish: Apply nail-polish remover with a glass rod, using the pad method. Sponge the remaining stain with denatured alcohol.

Paint: Scrape off fresh paint and wash in warm suds. If the stain has dried, soften first with oil, lard, or Vaseline. Then sponge with turpentine or banana oil. Wash in warm suds.

Perspiration: Wash in hot suds. Rinse. Bleach in the sun. If the stain remains, use hydrogen peroxide.

Shoe polish (wax): Sponge the spot with carbon tetrachloride. Launder. Treat any remaining stain with chlorine bleach. Rinse.

Sticky price tags: Spray with hairspray first, and if that doesn't work, apply nail-polish remover.

Sugar syrup: Wash in lukewarm soapy water.

Tea: For stains on cotten or linen, if they are fresh, treat as fruit stains. Or soak in borax solution (one teaspoon of borax to one cup of water), then rinse in boiling water.

Tobacco: Sponge with cold water. Work in warm glycerin. Let stand a half-hour. Or, if the stain is on cotton or linen, sponge with lemon juice or chlorine bleach.

Water: On silk, use a 5-percent solution of acetic acid. On velvet, hold the garment a few minutes over steam from a teakettle. Shake out until completely dry and brush.

For any spot or stain, if you are in doubt, consult your dry cleaner.

SPRAINS — Soak some coarse brown paper in cider vinegar and apply. Then cover with plastic.

Mix two cups of red clay soil with enough vinegar to thin it. Apply a heavy coat of this to the sprain and wrap with a towel or cloth.

Rub the sprain with a paste made of salt and the white of an egg.

Mix apple-cider vinegar with salt. Soak a cloth in this mixture and place the cloth on the injured area.

Stew a piece of alum the size of a walnut in the white of an egg until it forms a jelly. This should be placed over a sprain on a piece of lint.

Elevate your leg and apply cold compresses or an ice pack.

Try applying compresses of cold grated carrots.

SPROUTS — Sprouted seeds double their weight in three days. Sprouts are capable of sustaining life. Sprouts are also regenerating. One man wrote that sprouted oats restored fertility to sterile cattle. Now you'll want to know if this will work for people? In my opinion, it will in some cases.

Sprouts are easy to grow. Buy your seeds at a health-food store. Wash the seeds, put them in a jar and fill the jar with lukewarm water to stand overnight. The next day pour out the water and cover the jar with a paper towel held by a rubber band or with a screen lid, which makes washing the seeds easier. Rinse two or three times a day. Save the water for soups or juices or drink it. Next, lay the jar on its side by a warm window sill where it will get light. By the fourth day, tiny leaves and delicate tendrils will be bursting out of the jars. Sprouts are then easy to eat —roots, seeds, leaves, and all.

SQUIRRELS — To get rid of ground squirrels in the attic, mix cedar shavings with one-quarter cup of garlic powder and one-quarter cup of sulphur. Place in a plastic dish.

STAMMERING — Read aloud with your teeth closed for two hours each day for four months.

STATES — Eight states can be spelled using no more than four letters. They are: Alabama, Alaska, Hawaii, Indiana, Kansas, Mississippi, Ohio, and Utah.

STOCKS (BUYING) -- If you own stock, sell the day before a full moon. Then buy the third day after. Buy the fifth day before a new moon and sell the fifth day after.

Buy just before the last trading day of the month. Sell toward the end of the first nine days into the month. This does not apply for the month of February.

STOMACH PROBLEMS — Sick stomach: Take the inside of the bark of the slippery elm tree and make a powder and then a drink. It soothes and heals a sick stomach. Every part of the slippery elm is good for medicine—the leaves, berries, flowers, and bark.

Sour stomach: Chew a small piece of raw potato and swallow.

Stomachache: Drink Yerba Buena tea. It will taste like peppermint.

Stomach cramps: Drink ginger ale.

Stomach trouble: Make a tea out of remedies such as pagus (field marigold).

Drink blackberry juice.

Upset stomach: Take a medium-sized Irish potato and wash it off, but do not peel. Put the potato in a stew pan with water and let it cook. When it is done, take it out of the water and peel. Do not add any pepper, milk, or butter. Add just enough salt to get the potato down. The starch in the potato will soothe the lining of the stomach caused from vomiting so much. Soon your stomach is soothed down, and you feel better. Remember to use just enough salt to make the potato palatable. This is an old Indian herb remedy.

Take three sheets of unruled writing paper, the kind on which you write with ink and pen. Tear the pieces into little bits and put them in a glass of cool tap water. Let this stand for about fifteen or twenty minutes. Be sure all of the paper has gotten wet. Take the paper out of the glass of water and let the person with the upset stomach drink the water slowly. The gelatin that was on the tablet paper will settle the stomach. It is supposed to coat the lining of the stomach upset by too much vomiting.

Weak stomach: Beat some egg yolks and fresh mashed potatoes together and eat the mixture. Soon your stomach will be strong.

Eat clam broth.

STRESS — Try deep breathing and exercise to relieve stress.

Take up a hobby.

Talk out your problems.

Crying will help release tension.

Ten to twenty minutes of groaning (preferably while lying on the floor in a dark room) will help relieve stress.

Playing pleasant music will help you relax.

Vitamin C and iron supplements may help fight stress.

Make sure you get three hundred to four hundred milligrams of magnesium daily.

Sit or lie down. Close your eyes. Take a deep breath slowly. Exhale slowly. Imagine eating your favorite food.

STROKE — Eat a high-fiber diet.

Massage with olive oil or peanut oil.

Eat plenty of green vegetables.

Drink vegetable juices and soups.

Eat citrus fruits and drink their juices.

Avoid pork, red meats, and large amounts of starches.

You will need complete rest and relaxation.

STY — Tie a whole nutmeg around your neck and don't tell anyone. The sty will go away.

Put one or two drops of canned Pet milk in the eye.

Let a handful of fresh parsley steep for ten minutes in boiling water. Soak a cloth in the liquid, and then place it over your closed eye.

Bandage a tea bag (non-herbal) over your closed eye.

Rub the sty three times with a gold wedding ring.

SUGAR — Small children at the dining table can manage sugar easily if it is poured into a large salt shaker. Not only will it end spilling, but they'll use less.

You need much less sugar to give iced tea or coffee the desired sweetness if you dissolve the sugar in hot water before adding it to the tea or coffee. None will be wasted at the bottom of the glass or remain undissolved in the iced drink.

Hard brown sugar should be placed in a plastic bag with an apple that has been cut in six slices. Tie the bag so air cannot get in and place it in a slightly warm room. Within four hours the brown sugar should begin to crumble. Take out the apple slices. With the sugar still in the plastic bag, gently rub it between your hands.

SULPHUR — Use externally in skin cases, especially itching, in the form of ointment and as a vapor bath. Use internally on hemorrhoids, combined with magnesia as a laxative for children, and as diaphoretic in rheumatism. The dosage should be from one scruple to two drams mixed in milk or with treacle. When combined with an equal portion of cream of tartar, sulphur acts as a purgative.

SUNBURN — Sponge with vinegar. Let the vinegar dry, then take a warm shower. Most of the pain should be gone.

Wash the burned area with sour milk or buttermilk.

Rub with aloe-vera-leaf jelly.

Mix two tablespoons of vinegar in one-half cup of water, or mix equal parts of vegetable or olive oil and vinegar.

SWEATER (TO REMOVE FUZZ FROM) — Pull the sweater tightly over an ironing board. Shave lightly with a safety razor or use sandpaper.

S

SWEATS (NIGHT) — Stew two or three onions and eat them.

Drink plenty of cold sage tea.

Give a mixture of three parts salicylic and eighty-seven parts silicate of magnesia for sweating of the feet and night sweating by consumptives.

SWEETS (CRAVING FOR) — Mix the juice of two lemons with eight ounces of water. Drink this at 10:00 A.M. daily.

Drink one-half cup of Welch's grape juice at 10:00 or 10:30 A.M. and 3:30 P.M. each day.

When you feel that urge for sweets, place a clove in your mouth and gently suck on it. Do not swallow it. Leave it in the mouth for an hour.

The Fry-Son Sleeper

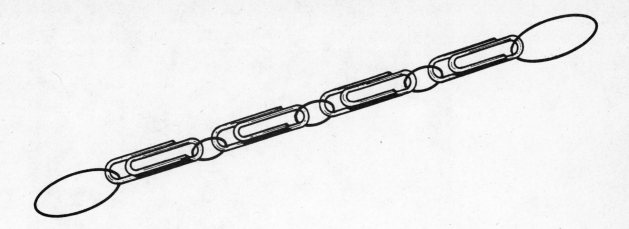

1. Get four paper clips, three very small rubber bands, and two normal-sized rubber bands.

2. Fasten the four paper clips with the three very small rubber bands.

3. On each outside paper clip, fasten one normal-sized rubber band.

4. Have a seat in your easy chair.

5. Place one outside rubber band over one thumb. Place the other outside rubber band over your other thumb.

6. Hold your arms straight in front of you.

7. Slowly begin to move each hand away from the other. Increase the speed of movement slowly.

8. Concentrate on the three small rubber bands.

9. After two minutes of doing this, you should be asleep.

10. The last thing you will remember before going to sleep is the three small rubber bands becoming one.

11. This does not work for everyone.

12. Some have said that this device will help cure the habit of biting your fingernails.

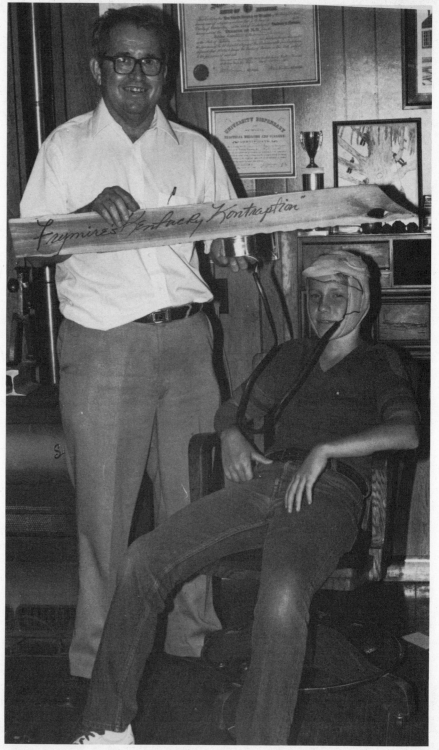

Fry's Scalp Stimulant

Dick and Troy try
out the device

Fry's Scalp Stimulant

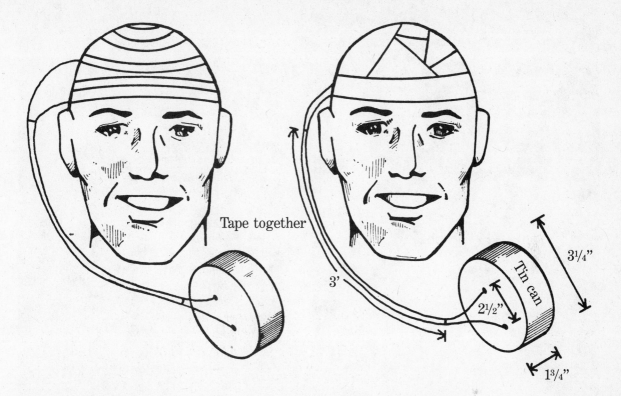

Tape together

3'

3¼"

Tin can

2½"

1¾"

1. Use two pieces of 14-gauge insulated copper wire nine feet in length.

2. Use one small tuna can to fasten the 14-gauge wire. (See illustration for where to bore holes and place bolts.)

3. Tape the two 14-gauge wires together, starting at the end of the can, three feet down. Then from the remaining six feet, strip insulation from the wire.

4. Beginning with the bottom six feet of wire, curl one piece as shown by the illustration. Place this circular piece on top of the head, securing it by using part of an Ace bandage.

5. Take the other six-foot piece of stripped wire and wrap it around the head above the ears. Then, use the remaining part of the bandage to hold it in place.

6. Rub a ¼" x 4" x 30" piece of wood edge-wise across the top of the can for approximately two minutes three times a day for ten days, then once a day for the next twenty days, then once every ten days.

7. Use this in conjunction with my baldness cure using onions (see page 12).

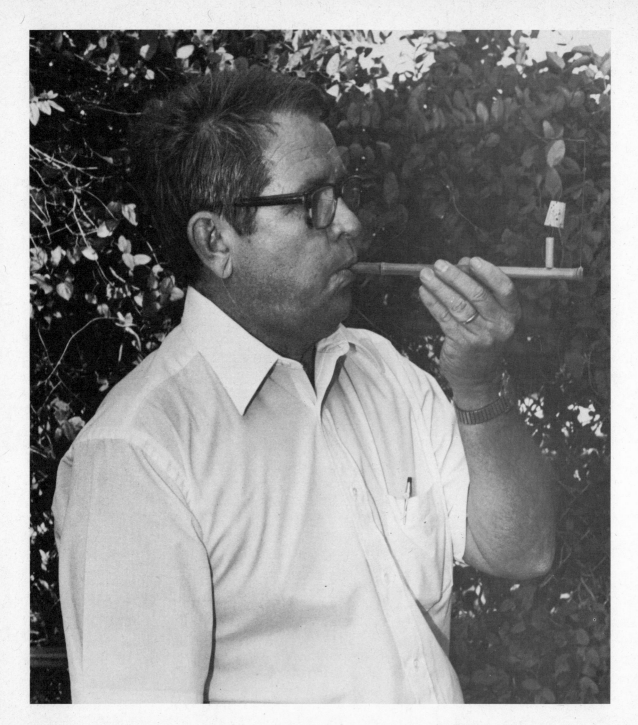

Frymire's Anti-Smoking Device

Anti-Smoking Device

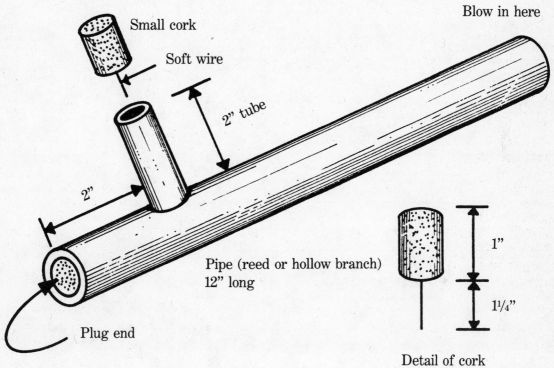

Small cork

Soft wire

2" tube

Blow in here

2"

Pipe (reed or hollow branch)
12" long

Plug end

1"

1¼"

Detail of cork
and soft wire

Blow into the reed to keep the cork aloft one-half inch for fifteen seconds. Do this every time you want a cigarette or at least thirty times a day.

You won't have time to smoke! That's one simple explanation for the miracle that the anti-smoking device can perform. Then, too, your lungs might not be able to handle a cigarette after so much blowing.

Hundreds have written to tell me that this works. Don't forget: follow the instructions.

*Former smokers—Tell Dick the story
of how you kicked the habit.*

_____

_____

_____

_____

_____

_____

_____

_____

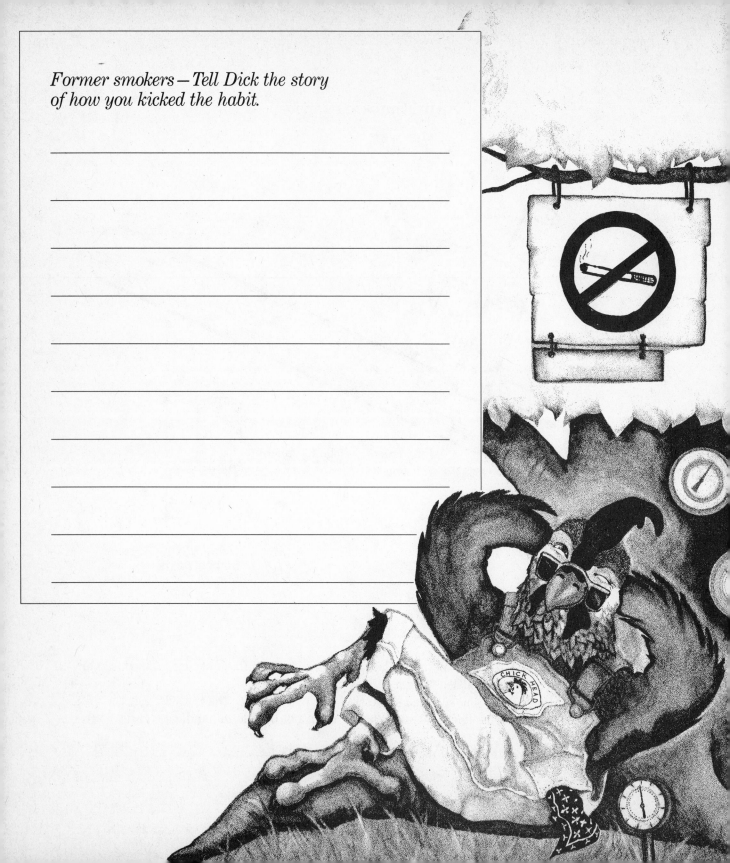

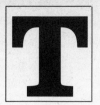

TABLE — Two card tables placed together won't move apart if strong rubber bands are slipped over adjoining legs.

TABLET (DENTURE) — Drop a denture tablet into the toilet, and it will help clean the bowl.

TARNISH (TO REMOVE FROM SILVER) — Use an aluminum pan or line a pan with aluminum foil. Use one cup of baking soda and mix it with two or three cups of water. Place the pan on the stove and bring to a boil. Take the pan off. Place silver in this mixture for ten minutes. Remove the silver and rinse. Good-by, tarnish.

Put camphor in a plastic bag with a soft cloth to clean silver trays and other larger items.

Put camphor balls in your silver chest.

TAR (TO REMOVE FROM SKIN) — Use Hellmann's mayonnaise to remove hot tar from skin.

TARTAR — To remove tartar deposit from the tongue side of the lower front teeth, mix two tablespoons of apple-cider vinegar with a glass of water. Sip this during meals.

TASTE (LOSS OF) — Eating foods rich in zinc can improve your sense of taste. Eggs, meat, seafood, liver, and dairy products are good natural sources of zinc.

TEETH — Brush your teeth twice a week with salt.

For clean teeth and fresh breath, break off the young asparagus-like shoots of the bright green meandering vine and eat them raw.

For sound teeth and gums, eat lettuce and raw carrots. Brush your teeth with a salt-and-soda mixture five times a week.

TEETHING — Rub the gums with olive oil.

Cut raw potato in thin slices and store the slices in the refrigerator in water. When needed, place one thin potato slice on your finger and gently rub the baby's gums.

TENDINITIS REMEDY — Place five drops of oil of wintergreen on one level teaspoon of baking soda. Put this in one-half glass of hot water (as hot as you can stand without scalding your throat). Stir and drink. Do this once a day for three days, and you could be one of the people that will never be bothered with tendinitis again. The oil of wintergreen is a poison, but the soda counteracts this oil. Don't forget to take this once a day for three days. It does not matter if you take it in the morning, afternoon, or night. It tastes a little like peppermint.

TENNIS BALLS — Have any of your tennis balls lost their zip? If so, wrap them in foil and bake them for twenty minutes in a two-hundred-degree oven. There will be more bounce to the ounce.

TENSION — Sip grape, apple, pineapple, or cherry juice at room temperature, not chilled. Some like to add an egg yolk to the cherry juice.

Chop an onion into small pieces and add one tablespoon of honey. Eat half with lunch and the other half with supper.

Eat a few strawberries (without cream and sugar) after each meal.

Drink warm peppermint tea.

Paint the walls of your room a light color.

Wear light blues and light grays.

Drink warm sage tea.

Mix three cups of Epsom salt with your bath water and soak for thirty minutes.

Eat celery.

TESTICLES (PAIN) — Massage the outer wrist of each hand and the outer ankle of each foot.

TETTER — A lady in Arkansas and another in Georgia had good results with the following: Mix two ounces of castor oil with just enough alcohol to cut the oil. Next add five drops of iodine. Mix well and apply to the affected area three times a day for ten days. You should be able to tell the difference by then.

Sometimes cucumber juice applied to the affected area will help.

Drink three ounces of apple juice twice a day.

THINGS YOU SHOULD KNOW — A man's total body weight is about 40 percent muscle. A woman's is about 30 percent.

The Old and New Testaments each contain the word *truth* exactly 117 times.

The heart of an elephant weighs forty-five pounds and would fill an ordinary bushel basket.

The earliest wristwatches date from 1790.

In one second, the sun sends out a million times more energy than is stored in all the earth's coal, petroleum, and natural gas fields.

The cat is the only domestic animal not mentioned in the Bible.

In a year your eyes move up and down and sideways some thirty-six million times. You blink them some eighty-four million times.

A person swallows about 585 times a day. The total includes 7.5 swallows an hour while sleeping, 36.5 an hour while reading, and the equivalent of 296 an hour while eating.

A female fox is called a vixen.

The difference between running and jogging is speed. A gait which has you going a mile in seven minutes or less is a run. A slower gait is a jog.

A piece of human skin as large as a postage stamp is said to contain three million cells, three feet of blood vessels, twelve feet of nerves, one hundred sweat glands, fifteen oil glands, and twenty-five nerve endings.

The American eel swims to the ocean to spawn; however, it lives and grows in fresh water.

There are 174,000,000 air cells in the lungs.

The world's shortest alphabet is Rotokas (South Pacific) with eleven letters. The longest is Cambodian with seventy-two.

The standard lead pencil contains enough graphite to draw a line thirty-five miles in length.

THISTLES (TO KILL) — Let them grow until they blossom, then cut them off near the top of the ground. The stalk will then be hollow. Water will get in the hollow and rot the stalks, so they will never sprout again. Do not cut below the ground.

THOUGHTS — For today's teenager, the key to happiness is the one that starts the family car.

Learn to love your enemies. Without them, you have no one to blame but yourself.

Women live longer than men because they have closets full of dresses they wouldn't be caught dead in.

This is a country of faith. On the installment plan you can buy what you can't afford. On the stock market you can sell what you don't own. On the tax form they take away what you haven't borrowed yet.

A generation ago, we were told we weren't as smart as our parents. Today, we are told we aren't as smart as our kids. Where, oh where, did we go wrong?

THROAT (INFECTION OR SORENESS) — Gargle with salt water—one-half teaspoon of salt to one-half cup of water.

Try drinking hot tea with honey.

Try mixing two tablespoons of vinegar and two tablespoons of honey in one-quarter cup of lemon juice. Heat and drink.

T

Use a candy sucker instead of a tongue depressor to check a child's throat.

Try tying a sock or scarf around your neck to keep it warm.

TICKS — To remove an embedded tick from your skin, let two drops of fingernail polish fall from the brush to cover the pest completely. In a few seconds, the tick will release its hold.

To remove a tick without pulling it off, rub Vick's salve on and around the tick, and it will turn loose.

Grasp the tick lengthwise with a pair of pointed tweezers, making sure the sharp end of the tool is right next to the skin, and once you've got a good hold on the tick, apply pressure and gently pull it off. If this pressure or procedure is done correctly, you'll probably remove a small piece of skin along with the whole tick. Be sure to destroy the tick. Wash the wound with soap and water, dry it off, and dab antiseptic on it. Then wash your hands.

A buried tick will back out intact if you cover it with petroleum jelly, alcohol, gasoline, or flea spray.

Drop a little mineral oil on a tick, and it will loosen its hold.

TINWARE — Never scour baking tins. They bake much better after they become brown.

To prevent rusting of tinware, rub it with beeswax.

TOADS — Toads are very useful as they live almost entirely upon slugs, caterpillars, beetles, and other insects. They make their rounds at night when we are asleep. Some people purchase toads and turn them loose.

TOE — Stub your toe. Kiss your thumb. Be very quiet and concentrate. You will be able to do things that you didn't think possible.

Fungus under the toenails: Squeeze a raw potato and apply the juice to the toenail three times daily for twenty days. You may have to chop the raw potato in very small pieces and place them in a cloth and squeeze. You should see an improvement by the end of the twenty days. At the end of that period, reduce treatments to twice daily.

Vitamin-E oil may also help.

Soak the foot in warm Epsom salt water for thirty minutes. Then take a firm brush and brush the nails.

In-grown nails: To cure, put a small piece of tallow in a spoon. Heat until the tallow becomes very hot, then pour it on the sore spot.

Tender toes: Soak feet in a strong tea solution twice daily for fifteen minutes. Let them dry. Apply castor oil. You should see results in ten to fourteen days.

TOLLABLE — If you are feeling just tollable, drink bitters tea made with whiskey, ratsbane, pokeberry, ginseng, and honey, plus sassafras, wild cherry, and slippery elm bark.

TOMATOES — Tomatoes, when eaten properly, are a good remedy for indigestion.

Pep up tomato juice by adding lemon juice and Worcestershire sauce. Serve icy cold in small glasses.

Wrap tomatoes (and apples) for storage with a cloth dipped in a solution of one pint of water to one tablespoon of chlorine bleach. Clean produce resists rot.

To keep tomatoes, cover with a solution of one teacup of salt to a gallon of water.

TONGUE (BURNED) — Rinse your mouth with cold water. Apply a few drops of vanilla extract.

TONIC — Eat persimmons and blackberries when they are ripe.

Mix two teaspoons of apple-cider vinegar (full-strength) with two teaspoons of local honey. Mix this combination with a cup of water. Begin by drinking this three times a day at mealtime for at least ten days. By the end of the tenth day, you should be getting that zing back. Just because you feel better, don't stop taking the tonic. Many have written to say that this tonic has helped their arthritis; others say it helps their allergies.

A good spring tonic is wild cherry bark tea.

Eat rhubarb once a week. Mix it with some sulphur and molasses and eat.

TONSILS — Your appendix and tonsils should not be removed unless it is absolutely necessary. They act as the focal point for poisons, gathering and sending them out through the proper channels.

TOOTHACHE — A small piece of cotton saturated with ammonia and placed next to a bad tooth will, in many cases, stop the aching.

Apply bruised or grated horseradish to the wrist.

To cure a toothache, drive a nail into an oak tree.

Place ice on the web of skin between the thumb and the index finger on the same side of the body as the toothache. This should help relieve the pain.

TOOTH (EXTRACTED) — An extracted tooth cavity packed with cotton wet with alum water will stop the bleeding.

TOOTH (POWDER) — Finely pulverized charcoal powder makes a good tooth powder.

TREES — Place crushed limestone around tree trunks to act as a shield against the tiny teeth of pine and meadow mice.

T

To tell the height of a tree, proceed from the base to a point where, on turning your back toward it and putting your head between your legs, you can just see the top of the tree. At the spot where you are able to do this, make a mark on the ground. Measure the distance from your mark to the base of the tree. This will be the tree's height.

Fruit trees will be safer if their trunks are painted white on the south side.

To protect fruit trees from mice, mix one part tar and three parts tallow. Apply hot to the bark of the tree with a paint brush.

Lime-washing your fruit trees while they are blossoming will drive the fruit pests away.

Do trees talk? Pick a time during the day, and every day for a week at that hour, go and sit under the tree and listen. Choose a tree that is in a quiet spot. Listen for fifteen minutes each time, and now you have the answer.

T-SHIRTS — Stretch old t-shirts over those old and frazzled bucket seats in your car or truck.

TURKEY — An old turkey has rough, reddish legs. A young turkey has smooth black legs. Fresh-killed turkeys' feet are moist.

TURNIPS — Turnip slices placed about your rosebeds will help control insects.

TURPENTINE — When turpentine is used to relieve pain or inflammation, it should be sprinkled on a piece of flannel that has been dipped in boiling water and wrung out as quickly as possible to preserve the heat.

TV SCREEN — Wipe your TV screen with a fabric softener paper and the glass will not attract dust.

TWITCHING AND SPASMS — Drink milk.

Sweeten with honey.

Massage the spine with olive oil.

Eat raw vegetables daily.

Avoid fried foods.

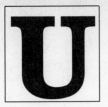

ULCER — Drink twelve ounces of raw, unfiltered, smelly cabbage juice twice a day for three months.

Do not drink coffee on an empty stomach.

URINARY PROBLEMS — Drink four cups of parsley tea a day.

Drink two cups of parsley juice daily.

Do not use soap, talcum powder, or colored or perfumed toilet paper on the genital area.

To heal kidney and bladder infections, drink one cup of cranberry juice at room temperature three times a day. Be sure the juice has no sugar or preservatives added.

To strengthen the kidneys and bladder, scrub a bunch of carrot tops and place them in one pint of boiling water. Let them steep for fifteen minutes. Drink three ounces of carrot-top water before each meal. After each meal, eat a handful of scrubbed celery tops. You should see a difference in three weeks.

To strengthen the bladder muscle, eat twenty-five unprocessed (unsalted) shelled pumpkin seeds three times a day.

To stimulate urination: Eat celery, watercress, parsley, watermelon, or raw cucumbers.
Drink corn-silk tea.
Grate one-half cup of horseradish and boil it with one-half cup of beer. Drink this mixture three times a day.

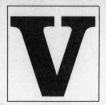

VAGINITIS — Always wear cotton panties. They will absorb moisture.

You should take showers instead of baths.

Do not use feminine hygiene sprays or other chemical products.

Do not wash panties with your other laundry. Wash them separately using a mild detergent and rinse them thoroughly.

Do not use colored toilet paper or tampons.

VARICOSE VEINS — Soak a piece of cheesecloth in witch hazel and wrap it around the infected areas.

Stand in a tub of cold water up to your knees for two or three minutes at the end of each day. Then walk briskly around the house for two or three minutes.

Wear support hose.

Elevate the legs frequently and try not to sit or stand for long periods of time.

Get plenty of exercise, such as walking, jogging, swimming, dancing, or cycling.

Lose weight if you are overweight.

Do not wear tight shoes.

VEGETABLES — Before slicing potatoes, dip your knife in boiling water to make them slice easier.

To keep vegetables from wilting, cut off the tops of carrots, beets, turnips, and parsnips before storing them.

Fried cucumber tastes somewhat like fried eggplant. Dip the slices in beaten egg and then dip them in bread crumbs. Fry until golden brown.

Place a one-inch square of bread on the point of your knife to absorb the fumes when you slice onions.

A piece of butter added to the water will keep vegetables from boiling over.

Bake a stuffed pepper or an apple in a muffin tin to keep its shape.

If you scorch vegetables, no one needs to know. Just set the pot in a pan of cold water and let it stand for twenty to thirty minutes. Don't scrape the bottom of the pot.

VINEGAR — At regular intervals pour boiling vinegar into kitchen drains to prevent grease blockage.

Vinegar boiled in a teakettle will remove sediment.

Plain vinegar is a very good water softener.

The best vinegar is made from special cider apples, which are processed with yeast. Let them ferment for four weeks and then age for six months.

VINES (GRAPE) — To prevent mildew, dust with sulphur and renew after each rain.

VITAMIN C — Eat wild violet blossoms, wild lettuce, lamb's quarters, dandelions, dock, purslane, and cattails. Either tossed in a salad or sauteed, they are healthful.

VOICE (TO RESTORE) — Beat the white of one egg and add the juice of one lemon. Sweeten with sugar. Take a teaspoon every half-hour.

VOWELS — Two words with all the vowels in the proper order are *facetious* and *abstemious*.

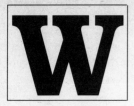

WALNUT (JUICE) — Crush the hulls of thirty walnuts. Place the crushed hulls in a five-gallon open container and cover with one gallon of water. Let the mixture stand for three days, stirring at least three times a day. At the end of the third day, strain the water off. This strained water is what I call walnut-hull juice.

WALNUT (TREE) — Walnut tree leaves are the last to leaf out each spring and the first to defoliate in the fall.

WAL-O-BLUE (FRYMIRE'S FISH-CATCH 'EM) — Mix one quart of walnut-hull juice, one-half cup of olive oil, and one teaspoon of clothes bluing. Place a little of this mixture on your live or artificial bait just before you cast the bait. Fish seem to be attracted to this mixture.

WARTS — During a full moon, cut a raw potato in half and rub it over the wart. Place the two halves together and bury them. When the potato rots, the wart will be gone.

Apply a used tea bag to the wart for fifteen minutes a day.

Drink eight ounces of camomile tea twice a day.

Use some soda with spirits of camphor. Apply to warts each evening.

Apply liquid vitamin E twice a day for two weeks.

Squeeze out the white milk of wild lettuce and rub it on the wart.

For warts on the genitals, rub the inside of a pineapple peel on the wart.

Twice a day put a mixture of grated carrots and one teaspoon of olive oil on the wart for one half-hour.

Twice a day apply lemon juice to the wart, then apply raw chopped onion for fifteen minutes.

Use the juice of the aloe vera plant.

Crush a fresh fig and apply it to the wart for one-half hour each day.

Mix castor oil and baking soda and apply.

Put the white, mushy side of a banana peel on the warts. There's a substance, a protein or an acid, that inhibits the ability of the virus within the wart to reproduce. The peel helps kill the wart, but not the surrounding skin. The banana peel softens the wart and the surrounding area, and later the bothersome growth can be clipped until it disappears. Be sure to tape the squishy side of the banana peel so that it covers the entire wart area. (This treatment also helps bunions and callouses.)

Rub warts with a bean leaf until they are green. They will soon disappear after a few applications.

Rub with glycerin.

Warm castor oil on gauze, applied three times a day for thirty minutes, should get rid of warts in three weeks.

Apply milkweed oil three times a day for four weeks.

Apply dandelion milk three times a day for three weeks.

At night, wash and dry a foot with warts. Apply apple-cider vinegar. Put a plastic bag over the foot and a sock over the bag. Rinse off in the morning. Repeat for as long as it takes for the warts to go away.

WASHING SOLUTION — Mix one gallon of warm water, one-half cup of white vinegar, one-half cup of ammonia, and one-quarter cup of baking soda. This is good for washing venetian blinds, woodwork, and painted walls.

WASPS — Foraging wasps, hornets, and yellow jackets hunt and kill a variety of destructive insects on garden vegetables and ornamentals. Like bees that pollinate plants, they should be appreciated as beneficial allies of the gardener.

Wasps, hornets, and yellow jackets don't leave stingers when they sting. If you get stung by one of these, apply a cold pack to the swollen area.

Wasps in the house can be quickly caught by using a water mister. The added weight on their wings makes them unable to fly.

Spray with alum water to get wasps out of buildings.

WATER — To determine whether water is safe to drink, put one-half pint in a clean bottle and add a few lumps of sugar. Tighten the lid on the bottle and place it in a warm, well-lighted room. If it remains clear after nine days of exposure, it is safe to drink. If it becomes murky, it is unsafe to drink.

Always boil water and let it cool before mixing it with food.

Hard water is any water that contains high amounts of calcium and magnesium. I believe hard water is much better for you than soft water.

Place two good-sized trout in your well to keep the water purified.

There are almost six hundred references to water in the Bible: for bathing and baptism, for washing of hands and feet, to cross, to conquer, in which to fish, to work by, and for being at peace. ("He leadeth me beside still waters. He restoreth my soul.")

W

Be sure to drink eight glasses of water a day. This will help clean out your system. In other words, water helps flush the wastes from your body through the most remarkable plumbing system ever invented.

WEEVILS (REMEDY) — Put several sticks of unwrapped spearmint gum on pantry shelves, and it will keep weevils out of flour. Put out fresh gum every three weeks.

WEIGHT (EASY LOSS METHOD) — Drink Welch's grape juice a half-hour before meals. It satisfies the body's craving for sugar and will break the habit of fattening desserts.

Much has been written on this subject. My conclusions are:
1) Eat less.
2) Exercise daily.
3) Eat slowly.
4) Try never to gain the first excess pound.
5) Keep busy.
6) Make a decision to lose.

WELD BURN (EYES) — Place a scraped raw potato on each eye.

Place raw potato juice in each eye.

WHIPPED CREAM — An egg white added to a cup of cream and beaten in with it will almost double the volume of whipped cream.

WHITE BREAD — White bread is perfectly wholesome if eaten in conjunction with an otherwise adequate diet of fruit, vegetables, and dairy products. So is cardboard!

WHITEWASH — Always mix skim milk with your lime to make the best whitewash.

WHOOPING COUGH — Breathe fumes of turpentine.

WINDOWS (TO CLEAN) — Combine one cup of cold water, one cup of rubbing alcohol, and one teaspoon of white vinegar. It would be best to use this in a spray-type container.

Use crumpled newspaper to clean windows instead of expensive paper towels.

Mix one quart of warm water, one-half cup of ammonia and one-eighth cup of white vinegar. This is especially good on mirrors.

WINE OR BEER — Elderly people should drink a glass or two of beer or wine daily. It is my opinion that they will be friendlier, more active, and happier. They will sleep better and complain less.

WOODENWARE — Clean woodenware immediately after use. Never immerse it in water or soak. Use as little water as possible. Keep it away from heat. Never place woodenware in the refrigerator. If woodenware is roughened, smooth it with sandpaper. Never polish, wax, or varnish it.

WOOL — To judge the quality of woolen material, squeeze it in your hand. It should feel smooth, rubbery, springy when you open your hand. If it has a rough feeling, the grade is inferior.

WORDS OF WISDOM — A lie has no legs to stand on, but it gets places.

Well begun is half done.

The human race has improved everything except people.

The devil can cite scripture for his purpose.

He who rides a tiger is afraid to dismount.

No wife can endure a gambling husband unless he is a steady winner.

When the fox cannot reach the grapes, he says they are sour.

Sympathy without relief is like mustard without beef.

Time heals all wounds and wounds all heels.

As a rule,
A man's a fool.
When it's hot,
He wants it cool.
When it's cool,
He wants it hot.
Always wanting, what is not.
— Author unknown

What goes over a sow's back comes under her belly.

Those who live beyond their means should act their wage.

A pound of honey represents the life work of about one thousand bees.

Insects suffer from many of the same kinds of diseases that human beings do.

The government rarely does something for you unless it does something to you.

The final six inches from success are between your ears.

The best labor-saving device is an inheritance.

Talk does not cook rice.

The man who wakes up and finds himself a success hasn't been asleep.

The art is not in making money but in keeping it.

Little expenses, like mice in a barn, when they are many, make great waste.

The average kiss uses up about nine calories. If you kiss 390 times, you will lose a pound.

Hair by hair, heads get bald.

A barrel is soon empty if but one drop a minute is lost.

If you mean to save, begin with your mouth.

Morals are caught, not taught.

If you want to know the meaning of the old adage "A fool and his money are soon parted," buy a lottery ticket.

You will soon get cold if you stretch your legs farther than the blanket will reach.

Any fool may make money, but it needs a wise man to spend it.

If you kick up dust, you are a poor worker.

If a man would have half his wishes, he would double his troubles.

Writing a will does not shorten a life.

The next time someone tells you nothing is impossible, ask him to dribble a football.

Two things are necessary for successful political campaigns: hot issues and cold cash.

When a little old lady sits at a spinning wheel these days, she's in Las Vegas.

Middle age is when the narrow waist and the broad mind begin to change places.

If you are too busy to pray, you are too busy!

When you point a finger at someone, you are pointing three at yourself.

By failing to prepare, you are preparing to fail!

Most people can keep a secret. It's the folks they tell it to who can't.

No matter what happens, there is someone who knew it would.

The best tranquilizer is a clear conscience.

WORMS — Bake the shell of one hen's egg until it turns brown and brittle. Crumble it up fine and mix the particles with honey and butter. Take every morning for a week.

To treat intestinal worms, chew some pumpkin seeds.

Drink elder-bark tea for parasitic screw worms.

WRENS — Wrens are called the people birds. It is good luck if a wren nests near your home. When a storm is near, wrens stay at home. They are valuable gardeners, for they feast upon insects, such as grasshoppers and beetles. They also snap up spiders, ticks, and plant life.

WRINKLED SKIN REMEDIES — To aid in bringing back that youthful look to skin, fix some cucumber juice. Wash parts of the body that are going to be massaged with the juice (usually the face). Let the area dry or pat it dry with a towel. Apply the juice with the hands and massage for five minutes. Let the massaged area dry. After it has been dry for thirty minutes, again wash all massaged areas with water, using a mild soap. Pat dry. Keep this up once a day for ten days. Then the juice should be applied and massaged in at least every two days. Store cucumber juice in the refrigerator. Your skin should get its youthful look back.

To make a mud pack, combine two cups of red clay soil with enough apple-cider vinegar to make a fine paste. Then add the white of one egg and mix well. Apply to the face. Let dry. Leave on for fifteen minutes. Crumble off. Wash with very mild soap. Rinse and pat dry.

Peel one fresh peach and take out the seed. Combine this and one cup of fresh cow's cream. Place the peach and the cream in a blender and mix. Massage the face with the mixture at least twice a day for ten days, then once a day thereafter. Massage for at least five minutes each treatment. You will like the results.

Mix some flour of sulphur in a little milk. Let it stand for three hours without disturbing. Use the milk as a lotion. Rub this lotion into the skin with a cloth. Wash the skin with a mild soap, rinse and pat dry.

Try a yogurt facial.

Eat a high-fiber diet.

Drink at least eight glasses of water each day.

Eat plums, apricots, blackberries, and green peppers, especially the velvety white inner fibers and seeds.

Eat almonds.

Season food with garlic.

Drink buttermilk.

Rub wrinkles with castor oil.

Mix three ounces of castor oil with just enough alcohol to cut the oil. Then add the juice of one-half of a ripe peach. Massage wrinkles for five minutes. Repeat again in ten minutes. Now, very gently, wash the area with a very mild soap. Rinse and pat dry. Do this treatment each day for thirty days. If you like the results, continue on every other day.

Drink some bird-grape wine. The small, wild grape known to boys as the "bird grape" never attains it full sweetness until after the fall of frost. It makes an excellent wine for culinary purposes. This kind of grape must be used in your wine-making if you wish to improve your skin condition. Drink at least three ounces per day.

Drink at least two cups of wild grape juice a day.

W

Mix equal parts of brewer's yeast and yogurt. Apply, let dry, wash off.

Boil one-half cup of milk, two teaspoons of lemon juice, and one tablespoon of brandy. Apply warm, let dry, wash off with lukewarm water.

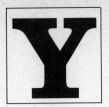

YELLOWROOT TEA — Drink yellowroot (*Xanthorhiza simplicissima*) tea for sore mouth, sore eyes, and stomach trouble. Many people take it for ulcers. Make it by putting one-half cup of yellowroot in a quart of water and boiling it for thirty minutes.

YOGURT — Just what is it? Yogurt is fermented milk. Some say it will make hair grow; some eat it and use it for facials; some say it is associated with sexual prowess and a cure-all for about anything. Some say it is the milk of life.

Yogurt is especially good for disturbances of the intestinal tract. Some say it has been found to be a tumor retardant. Some say it cures diarrhea quicker than drugs. People who can't tolerate milk because they lack the proper enzyme to handle its lactose can enjoy and benefit from natural lactobacillus yogurt.

There are many good books that tell you how to make yogurt. You will find that it is not hard to make, but I also know that most of you will buy the store-bought kind.

Acne 1
Acne (Scars) 1
Age (Guess) 2
Age (Spots) 2
Alcohol (Breath) 2
Alcohol (Cleaner) 2
Alcoholism 2
Ale (Rhubarb) 2
Alfalfa 2
Allergies 2-3
Aloe 3
Aluminum Foil 3
Anemia 3
Angina Pectoris 3-4
Animal Remedies 4
Anti-Smoking Device 168-169
Ants 4-5
Appendicitis 5
Apples 5
Arteries (Hardening) 5-6
Arthritis 6-9
Artichoke (Jerusalem) 9
Asparagus 9
Asthma 9-10
Athlete's Foot 10

Baby (Baby Food That Can Be
    Digested When All Else Fails) 11
Baby (Potion to aid in resting) 11
Back Pain Zapper 25
Back Problems 11-12
Baking (Hints) 12
Baldness 12-13
Banana Bread 13
Barley 14
Basement Dampness 14
Basil 14
Bathing (Rules) 14

Beads 14
Beans (Baking) 14
Beauty Treatments 15
Bed Bugs 15
Bed Sores (To Prevent) 15
Bed Wetting 15
Beef (To Corn) 15-16
Beekeepers 16
Bee Sting (To Relieve) 16
Beets 16
Biliousness (Remedy for) 16
Birds 16
Birth 16-17
Bites and Stings (Insects) 17
Blackberry Pickers 17
Blackheads 17
Bladder (Infection) 17
Bleeding (How to Stop) 17
Blight (Fruit Trees) 17
Blindness (Night) 17
Blood (Clots) 18
Blood (Fortifiers) 18
Blood (Low, Remedy) 18
Blood Pressure (High) 18-19
Blood Pressure (Low) 19
Blossoms (Flower) 19
Blues 19
Body Weakness and Exhaustion 19
Boils 19
Bone (Protection) 20
Bone Meal (As Protection from
    Potato Bugs) 20
Borers (To Protect Trees from) 20
Bottles (Clean) 20
Bowles (To Regulate) 20
Box (Measures) 20
Brain (Stimulate) 20
Bran 20
Brass and Copper (To Clean) 20

Bread (Hints) 20-21
Breast (Problems) 21
Breath (Bad) 21
Bronchitis 21-22
Broom (Tips) 22
Bruises 22
Brushes (Paint) 22
Buckeye 22
Bunion (Cure) 22
Burns 22-23
Bursitis 23-24
Butter (To Color) 24
Buttermilk 24
Buttermilk (As a Cleanser) 24
Buttons (To Remove) 24

Cabbage (Grubs) 27
Cabbage (Made Digestible) 27
Cabbage (Red) 27
Cake 27
Calamus (Root) 27
Calcium 27-28
Calcium (Deposits) 28
Camomile 28
Campers (Tips) 28
Canaries (Care of) 28-29
Cancer 29
Cancer (Lung) 29
Cancer (Old-Time Cure) 29
Cancer (Skin) 29
Candle 29-30
Canker and Cold Sores 30
Carpet (To Restore Faded) 30
Carrots 30
Castor Oil (Hot Packs) 30
Cataracts (To Help Prevent) 30
Catnip 30
Cats' Problems 31

Cauliflower 31
Cayenne Pepper 31
Celery 31
Cereal 31
Chair (Cane-Bottomed, to Restore) .. 31
Chamois (Stiff) 32
Cheese 32
Chest (Congestion) 32
Chicken Pox 32
Chickens 32-33
Chigger (Bites) 33
Child Training and Problems
    with Behavior 33
Chills 33
Chimney (Clean) 33-34
Chimney Lamp (How to Clean) 34
China 34
Chips (Keep Fresh) 34
Cholesterol (High) 34
Cigarette (Smoke) 34
Circulation (Problems) 34
Cirrhosis 34-35
Clean (House) 35
Cleansing Cream 35
Clock (Soundproof) 35
Clothespins 35
Clothing (Care of) 35-36
Coat (Fur) 36
Cockroaches 36
Coconut 36
Coffee 36
Colds 36-38
Colic 38-39
Colitis 39
Colon (Stopped Up) 39
Color Blindness 39-40
Combs (Clean) 40
Complexion 40
Constipation 40-41

Consumption 41
Convulsions 41
Cooking (Hints) 41
Corks (Enlarging) 41
Corn (Cooking) 41
Corn (Earworm) 41
Corn (Planted) 42
Corns 42
Coughing 42-43
Cow 44
Cow (Tea) 44
Cow (Utter Caked) 44
Cradle Cap 44
Cramp (While Bathing or Swimming) ... 44
Crayon (Marks, Removing
    from Painting Walls) 44
Crickets 44
Crops (Estimate) 44-45
Crops (Harvest) 45
Croup (Krup) 45
Cucumber Vines 45
Curtains (To Mend) 45
Cuts and Wounds 45-46
Cutworms 46
Cysts 46

Daisies 47
Dandelions 47
Dandruff 47
DDT 47
Decongestant 47
Defroster 48
Dental Problems 48
Deodorizer 48
Depression 48
Diabetes 48-49
Diamond (To Test Authenticity) 49
Diaper (Pins) 49

Diaper Rash 49
Diarrhea 49
Diets 49-50
Diets (Frymire's Potato) 50
Diplodia (Twig Blight) 50
Digestive Problems and Nausea 50
Diseases (Childhood, Treatment of) ... 50-51
Disinfectants 51
Dizziness 51
Dog 51
Dog Days 51
Dog Problems 51-52
Doughnuts 52
Dowsing 52
Drain (Prevent Clogging) 52
Drain Cleaner 53
Drinker (Social) 53
Dropsey 53
Dysentery 53

Ear (Noises) 54
Ear (Problems) 54
Ear (Ringing) 54-55
Ear (Trouble: Infection and
    Wax Build-up) 55
Earache 55
Eczema 55-56
Eggs 56
Emotional Problems 56
Etiquette (Table) 56-57
Exercise (For Your Back) 57
Eyes 57-58

Face (Clean) 59
Face (Shave) 59
Fainting 59
Faithfulness 59

Fatigue 59
Faucets 59
Feet 59-60
Female Problems (Frigidity) 60
Fence Post (To Keep from Rotting) 61
Fertility (Remedy) 61
Fever 61
Fever Blisters 61-62
Fever (Drink) 62
Fever (Hay) 62
Figs 62
Fingernails 62
Fish 62-63
Fish-a-lex Attractor 71
Fishing (Trip) 63
Fits (Treatment for Those
    Caused by Indigestion) 63
Fleas (In House) 63
Flies (To Destroy) 63
Flour 63
Flowers (Cut) 63-64
Flu 64
Forecasting 64-69
Fortune 69
Fountain 69
Fountain of Youth 69
Foxglove 69
Freckles (To Remove) 69
Freezes 69
Frostbite 69
Fruit Rolls 69
Frymire Fish Finder and Attractor 72
Frymire's Weather Service
    and Museum 73-74
Fry-Son Sleeper 165-166
Fumigate (Home) 70
Funnel 70
Furniture (To Clean) 70
Furniture (Polish) 70

Furniture (Scratches) 70

Gall Bladder (Problems) 75
Galls (Harness or Saddle) 75
Game 75
Garden Tips 75-76
Garden Tools 76
Garlic 76-77
Gas 77
Geese 77
Ginseng 77
Glassware 77
Gold Chains (To Clean) 77
Goldenrod 77
Goldenseal 77-78
Gout (Cure) 78
Gout Pain Reliever 79
Greens 78
Ground Hog 78

Hair 81-82
Hands (Brown Spots) 82
Hands (Cleaner) 82
Hands (Perspiring) 82
Hands (Rough) 82
Hands (Soft) 82
Handshake 82
Hangover 82-83
Harvest Drink 83
Head 83
Head Noise 83
Headache Remedies 83-86
Health (Hints) 86-88
Heart (Pain) 88
Heart (Strengthen) 88
Heart (Weak) 88
Heartburn 88

Heating Pad 88
Hemorrhoids 88-89
Hens 89
Herbs 89
Hernia 89
Herpes 89
Hiccups 89
Hives 90
Hoarseness 90
Hole (Dig) 90
Hole (In Screen) 90
Home (Before Buying) 90
Honey 90
Hoosier 90-91
Horse (Balky) 91
Hot Flashes 91
Horseradish 91
Household Hints 91-95
Hunters 95
Hydrangeas 95

Iceburgs 97
Icehouse 97
Ice Idea 97
Impotence and Sexual Problems 97-98
Indigestion 98-99
Inflammation 99
Ink Stain 99
Insect Bites and Stings 99-100
Insect Repellents 100
Insecticide (Critter
   Ridders and More) 100-103
Insomnia 104-105
Intestinal Fever 105
Intestinal Problems 105
Iron Deficiency 105
Irons (To Smooth) 105
Itch (Bug Bites) 105

Itch (Jock) 105
Itch (Rectal) 106

Jaundice 107
Jelly Molds 107
Jelly Testing 107
Jewelry (To Clean) 107
Jewelweed 107

Kentucky Kontraption 111-112
Keys (Piano) 108
Kidney Problems 108
Kitchen Hints 108-110
Knees (Knock) 110
Knives (Care of) 110

Ladybugs 113
Lamps (To Prevent Smoking) 113
Lawn Mowing 113
Leather (To Soften) 113
Leaves 113
Legs (Cramps) 113
Legs (Pain) 113
Legs (Shaving) 113
Lemons 114
Lend 114
Lice 114
Lice (Hens) 114
Liniment (For Man or Beast) 114
Lips 114
Liquids 115
Lockjaw (Treatment for) 115
Locks (How to Fits Keys to) 115
Lore 115
Lunar (Month) 115
Lungs 115-116

Malaria 117
Man 117
Mange 117
Marble 117
Maypop 117
Measure (Land) 117
Measure (Liquid) 117
Meat (Economy in) 117-118
Medical Hints 118
Medicine 118
Memory (Improving) 118
Memory (Loss) 118
Men (How to Judge) 119
Menopause 119
Menstrual Problems 119
Mental Problems 119
Mice 120
Mildew 120
Milk 120
Milkweed 120
Mirror (Steaming) 120
Miscellaneous 120-122
Mistletoe 123
Moles (Body) 123
Moles (Underground) 123
Money Maxims 123
Mood Rhythms 123
Moon 123
Moon and Zodiac Signs 124
Moons (Signs) 124-125
Morning Sickness 125
Mosquito Zapper 127-128
Moss (On Trees) 125
Moths 125
Motion Sickness 125
Mouth 125-126
Muffins 126
Mumps 126
Mush (Fried Cornmeal) 126

Mushrooms 126

Nap 129
Nature 129
Nausea 129
Neck (Enlarged) 129
Neck (Stiff) 129
Nerve (Pinched) 129
Nervousness 129-130
Neuralgia 130
Nipples (Sore) 130
Nose (Shiny) 130
Nose Bleeds 130-131

Obesity 132
Odor (Body) 132
Odor (Car) 132
Odor (Cooking) 132
Odor (Fish) 132
Odor (Foot) 132
Odor (Refrigerator) 133
Odor (Smoke) 133
Odor (Turnips) 133
Oil Paintings 133
Ointment 133
Old Way of Saying Something 133
Olives 133
Onion (Bags) 133
Onion (Breath) 133
Onions 133
Oranges 133-134
Ornaments 134
Osage Orange 134
Osteoporosis 134
Oysters (Imitation) 134

Pain 135

Paint 135
Papered Walls (To Clean) 135
Parchment (To Treat Paper) 135
Parsley 135
Patent Leather 136
Patina (To Obtain) 136
Pears 136
Peas 136
Pesticide 136
Phlebitis 136
Photographs 136
Pick-Me-Up Drink 136
Pie 136
Pigeons (Homing) 136
Pill (Swallowing) 136
Pillow (Down) 136
Pimples 137
Pineapple 137
Pinworms 137
Plants 137-138
Plate (Cracked) 138
Poison Ivy 138-139
Poisons (To Drive Out) 139
Pokeweed 139
Popcorn 139
Potatoes 139
Potatoes (A Treat) 139
Potatoes (Sweet) 140
Pregnancy 140
Premenstrual Tension 140
Products (Natural) 140
Prostate Problems 140
Psoriasis 140-141
Puff (Powder) 141
Pulmonary (Complaints) 141
Pumpkin (Seeds) 141
Putty (To Remove from Windows) 141
Pyorrhea 141

Questions 142-143
Quinsy 143

Rabbit Tobacco 144
Rain Machine 147-148
Raisins 144
Rashes 144
Rats (To Exterminate) 144
Records (Warping) 144
Fry-Hut Relaxer 149-150
Remedies 144-145
Rheumatism 145
Ribbon (To Clean) 145
Rice 146
Ring (Collar) 146
Ringworm 146
Roach Ridder 146
Roofing Mix 146
Rope (To Soften) 146

Salt 151
Salve (Black) 151
Salve (White) 151
Sassafras 151
Sauerkraut 151
Scalp (Dry) 151-152
Fry's Scalp Stimulant 167
Scarlet Fever (Treatment) 152
Scars 152
Sciatica (Leg and Back Pain) 152
Sciatica (Sore Hip) 152
Scissors (To Sharpen) 152
Scratches (To Cure) 152
Screw (To Loosen) 152
Scrotum and Testicles 152
Sea Sickness (Sure Preventative) 152
Sea Sickness (Treatment) 152-153

Sedative (Mild) 153
Seeds 153
Self-Control 153
Sewer Pipes 153
Sewing Hints 153
Shampoo (Rug) 153
Sheet-Iron Stove (To Preserve) 153
Shingles 153-154
Shoes 154
Signs 154
Silverware 154
Sinus (Trouble) 154-155
Skin Problems 155-156
Slugs 156
Smoking 156
Snacks 156
Snails 156
Snakes (Under House) 156
Sneezing 156
Snowdrift Remedy 156
Soaking (Clothing) 156
Soap Making 156
Sock 156
Soda (Baking) 157-158
Soda (Low-Calorie) 158
Sodium (Lowering Intake) 158
Soil (To Test) 158
Some Things To Know 158
Sores and Burns 158
Sore Spot 158
Sore Throat 159
Soups 159
Spots and Stains (To Remove) 159-161
Sprains 161
Sprouts 161
Squirrels 161
Stammering 161
States 161
Stocks (Buying) 161

Stomach Problems 161-162
Stress 162
Stroke 162-163
Sty 163
Sugar 163
Sulphur 163
Sunburn 163
Sweater (To Remove Fuzz from) 163
Sweats (Night) 164
Sweets (Craving For) 164

Table 171
Tablet (Denture) 171
Tarnish (To Remove from Silver) 171
Tar (To Remove from Skin) 171
Tartar 171
Taste (Loss of) 171
Teeth 171
Teething 171
Tendinitis Remedy 171-172
Tennis Balls 172
Tension 172
Testicles (Pain) 172
Tetter 172
Things You Should Know 172-173
Thistles (To Kill) 173
Thoughts 173
Throat (Infection or Soreness) 173-174
Ticks 174
Tinware 174
Toads 174
Toe 174
Tollable 174
Tomatoes 175
Tongue (Burned) 175
Tonic 175
Tonsils 175
Toothache 175

Tooth (Extracted) 175
Tooth (Powder) 175
Trees 175-176
T-shirts 176
Turkey 176
Turnips 176
Turpentine 176
TV Screen 176
Twitching and Spasms 176

Ulcer 177
Urinary Problems 177

Vaginitis 178
Varicose Veins 178
Vegetables 178
Vinegar 179
Vines (Grape) 179
Vitamin-C 179
Voice (To Restore) 179
Vowels 179

Walnut Juice 180
Walnut (Tree) 180
Wal-O-Blue
  (Frymire's Fish-Catch Em') 180
Warts 180-181
Washing Solution 181
Wasps 181
Water 181-182
Weevils (Remedy) 182
Weight (Easy Loss Method) 182
Weld Burn (Eyes) 182
Whipped Cream 182
White Bread 182
Whitewash 182

Whooping Cough 182
Windows (To Clean) 182
Wine or Beer 182
Woodenware 182-183
Wool 183
Words of Wisdom 183-184
Worms 184
Wrens 184
Wrinkled Skin Remedies 185-186

Yellowroot Tea 187
Yogurt 187

Special requests for forecasts for events such as fairs, family reunions, picnics, festivals, weddings, car or horse races, golf tournaments, etc., are accepted. Requests should be made at least four months in advance in order to forecast accurately. Six months in advance allows for an even more accurate forecast.

For the special date or dates, I will need the longitude and latitude and elevation of the particular location.

A fee for special forecasting is required, as is a stamped, self-addressed envelope for reply to all correspondence. If at all possible, I answer every letter and special request personally. General snow forecasts are available September 1, and the wet-dry forecast is available March 15. Special events forecasts are available any time, as long as the suggested lead time (above) is possible.

In addition to the weather forecasting service, I operate a small museum on the lot next to the weather tree. All my folklore inventions are on display there, and visitors have the opportunity to see Fred the Rabbit, Zeb the Skunk, Oscar and Rosemary the Cowsucker Snakes, and, of course, Ted the Rooster and his lovely wife, Miss Maudie.

Please direct all inquiries to: Dick Frymire, c/o Frymire Weather Service, 314 North Chestnut Street, P.O. Box 33, Irvington, Kentucky 40146. My partners are my son, J. L. Frymire, and my grandson, Troy Jones.

If you have remedies or pieces of wisdom you would like to share with us and with readers of future editions, please write to us at the address above.